Passing the ARC

Successful portfolio-based learning

Passing the ARCP

Successful portfolio-based learning

By Samuel P. Dearman, Adam B. Joiner,
Samantha Abbott and Damien Longson

RCPsych Publications

© The Royal College of Psychiatrists 2014

RCPsych Publications is an imprint of the Royal College of Psychiatrists,
21 Prescot Street, London E1 8BB
http://www.rcpsych.ac.uk

British Library Cataloguing-in-Publication Data.
A catalogue record for this book is available from the British Library.
ISBN 978 1 909726 20 8

Distributed in North America by Publishers Storage and Shipping Company.

The views presented in this book do not necessarily reflect those of the Royal College of
Psychiatrists, and the publishers are not responsible for any error of omission or fact.

Printed by Bell & Bain Limited, Glasgow, UK.

Contents

Authors

Dr Samuel P. Dearman is now a consultant psychiatrist in working-age adult services in Cumbria as well as Director of Medical Education, but began this book during year 6 specialty training (ST6). He was a student at the University of Manchester at the undergraduate and postgraduate level. He has been involved in research in mental health legislation, epidemiology and evidence-based service provision, and has published in peer-reviewed journals. He has a special interest in education and has been involved in a variety of projects integrating contemporary learning theory into individual, team-based and organisational learning as well as the delivery of mental health training to psychiatric trainees, mental health service staff and other professionals outside mental health.

Dr Adam B. Joiner is currently working as an ST5 in general adult psychiatry in the North West. He completed his undergraduate medical degree at King's College London, where he also intercalated a BSc in neuroscience and neuropsychology. He has done psychiatry training in North West England, throughout Lancashire and Cumbria. He has been involved in medical education throughout training and is currently completing the postgraduate diploma in medical education before undertaking a Masters in medical education. He sits on the council for Manchester Medical Society's Section of Psychiatry.

Mrs Samantha Abbott is the medical education manager for the North Western Deanery School of Psychiatry, supporting and coordinating training for 250 trainees, from Cheshire to Cumbria. He has a background in business studies and has overseen the design, implementation and support for the first psychiatry e-portfolio in the UK. She has also built strong expertise in helping trainees manage their portfolios and prepare for the anual review of competence progression (ARCP).

Dr Damien Longson is the Head of School of the North Western Deanery School of Psychiatry, a consultant liaison psychiatrist and an active member of several education committees at the Royal College of Psychiatrists. He also chairs all the psychiatry ARCPs for the North Western Deanery. After doing basic training in medicine and psychiatry, he received a Wellcome Foundation Research Scholarship and studied the glutamate hypothesis of schizophrenia for a PhD in California and Boston, USA, before becoming a senior trainee in Manchester, UK.

Figures, boxes and tables

Foreword

Professor Jacky Hayden CBE

I was delighted to be invited to write the foreword for this book, which I hope will encourage many trainees to approach their learning with greater understanding and present themselves in the best light at the annual review of competence progression (ARCP).

Knowing how to maintain a portfolio as a useful record of learning and reflection can be difficult for any doctor new to specialty training, and understanding how to demonstrate learning through the portfolio to present at the ARCP can be particularly challenging. This slim volume describes the importance of collecting and collating information about a doctor's experiences so that the portfolio will easily demonstrate that the competencies expected for that period of training have been completed. It outlines the importance of reflection and how to write reflectively so that learning can be achieved and retrieved from daily experiences, and how to present materials in a logical manner. Chapter 3 is written as an interview with two key figures in the school of psychiatry in one deanery. Together, the interviewer, the head of school and the medical education manager describe how they use the information presented to them to judge whether or not a trainee is making adequate progress. The style enables the authors to identify many of the pitfalls for trainees approaching their ARCP.

This book will aid any medical trainee in their ARCP preparation and will be particularly useful for those training in psychiatry.

Preface

When we first decided to write this book, I was enthused and optimistic that we should be able to set out a framework for putting together a developmental portfolio that is logical and informative for the benefit of all psychiatric trainees, and indeed trainers. As a group, we want to pool perspectives and experience from training, administration and the ARCP panel, bringing together a coherent set of guiding principles. When I was a trainee, I often wondered whether the portfolio was a friend or an enemy. It is accepted that the portfolio, and ultimately the ARCP, requires a huge amount of work by trainees in terms of time, effort and planning. The successful portfolio can represent physical evidence of development over time, abilities and achievements. Equally, however, the portfolio is a source of anxiety and uncertainty for many trainees, especially when it comes to the ARCP. One of the difficulties is that there is no 'right' way to demonstrate competence and guidance has been sketchy. It is for these reasons that I am confident that this book is a useful guide for all trainees throughout their years in specialty training as well as being a reference material for trainers and educational supervisors.

Dr Samuel P. Dearman

Acknowledgements

We would like to thank the following people for their help and support: Professor Else Guthrie, Joanne Waddington, Dr Andrew Morgan, Karen March and Leanne Dearman.

Abbreviations

ACE   Assessment of Clinical Expertise
ARCP   annual review of competence progression
CbD   case-based discussion
CCT   Certificate of Completion of Training
CRHT   crisis resolution and home treatment
CPD   continuing professional development
CT   core trainee/training
CV   curriculum vitae
DONCS   Direct Observation of Non-Clinical Skills
GMC   General Medical Council
GP   general practitioner
ILO   intended learning objective
LETB   local education and training board
mini-PAT   mini Peer Assessment Tool
NHS   National Health Service
PDP   personal development plan
ST   specialty trainee/training
WPBA   workplace-based assessment

How to use this guide

This book is a guide and not a set of rules – there will be alternative approaches to organising and populating a portfolio. Across the UK different programmes will use different portfolios, in paper or electronic versions, allowing varying amounts of freedom in terms of structure and presentation. Throughout this book there are repeated references to planning, assessment, reflective practice, development and evidence. This is intentional, reminding the reader of the guiding principles underlying the successful negotiation of the ARCP. There is an emphasis on using the portfolio as a tool that catalogues evidence and drives learning, and because the portfolio will change and improve over time, some educationalists refer to it as a living document. However, it is equally important that the portfolio is readable and well structured.

The first chapters of this book provide the reader with an insight into the background of the present approach to psychiatric training and how the portfolio fits into this. Included are lessons learned following the first years of specialty training and the ARCP process, which includes perspectives from training, administration and the ARCP panel. The book then looks at the individual sections of the psychiatric training portfolio in some detail. Each chapter, as far as possible, aims to follow the same structure such that trainees can translate its content into a method of using the portfolio to communicate evidence of competence effectively. Chapters begin with basic principles, often followed by bullet points in the form of prompts or questions. The methods suggested are then applied to specific examples, where possible comparing good and less successful practice. Because there is no 'right' way to produce the portfolio, the hope is to illustrate the issues early in each chapter by use of examples and not simply to spoon-feed directives. Trainees can apply the basic principles and prompts to see why the examples are informative, or uninformative, and then use this as a framework to structure their own work.

If this book helps trainees develop a conceptual framework as to how to plan their learning according to curriculum competencies and structure their portfolio to follow training, making each section logical and informative, then it has achieved its goal.

CHAPTER 1

Quick reference guide

The portfolio

- The successful portfolio is a developmental tool that builds a collection of evidence of experience, assessments of competence, self-reflection and personal development planning over time.
- Trainees should 'own' the portfolio by managing their own learning, using the portfolio as an iterative tool.
- Portfolio evidence of competence must demonstrate trainees' performance in reality rather than their factual knowledge or abilities in controlled examinations.
- Evidence of achievement of competencies occurs by combining different forms of evidence and assessments in various contexts and with multiple assessors.
- The more often the portfolio is used, the better, using formal points of appraisal as landmarks.
- True evidence in the portfolio is clear, transparent and demonstrable proof of competence.
- The evidence should not be overstretched.
- Attending a training course is not in itself evidence of competence.
- The portfolio supports the General Medical Council (GMC) revalidation process (General Medical Council, 2013).

Organising the portfolio

- Organisation and reference to clearly indexed, triangulated evidence at the start of the portfolio sets the tone.
- Make it user-friendly; summarise evidence and clearly state the competency, giving clear and specific locations of evidence.
- How much is enough evidence? Two sources at least and three where possible.
- Plan your educational objectives early with reference to competencies.
- Remember that 'if it is not documented, it did not happen'.

- Do not breach confidentiality within the portfolio. Never use patient-identifiable material. If letters about patients are included, remove all identifiers.
- Do not leave portions of the curriculum uncovered, especially if they are hard to evidence. Consider mapping the gaps.

Workplace-based assessments (WPBAs)

- The need to evidence a particular competence should drive which WPBA is chosen, not the other way round. Workplace-based assessment should occur regularly throughout a period in training. Do an Assessment of Clinical Expertise (ACE) early on as a benchmark.
- Present WPBAs in a logical sequence with a clear description of the experience and associated competencies.
- Link WPBA to reflective practice and show how this informs your professional development.
- Capitalise on opportunities in routine work – if you are discussing a case as a part of daily work, use it as a case-based discussion (CbD) WPBA.
- Patient feedback can be a powerful driver for learning. It comes in many forms and should be used even when it is challenging (e.g. complaints, thank-you letters, cards as well as formal feedback tools).

Reflective practice

- Reflective practice is a process of learning and development through focusing on thoughts and feelings.
- The successful portfolio must contain a good amount of reflective practice relating to both clinical and non-clinical experience.
- Reflective notes should cover the nature of the experience, any feedback, lessons learned and how these inform professional development.
- Trainees must decide how to make reflective notes more informative, by either filing them in a separate section of the portfolio or filing them where relevant, or a combination of these approaches.

Audit and research

- As a starting point, check early on exactly what competencies you need to evidence – planning is key.
- Not everybody will do a full-blown research project, but you must make sure you meet the requirements of your curriculum.
- For trainees with projects, present these in brief and then in detail if appropriate, making it clear what your skills are and what your involvement in the project was.

- If you have been involved in research, some academic skills can be evidenced in a variety of ways including simple approaches such as journal clubs.

Teaching

- Presentation of teaching experience should describe the task, topics, teaching methods, skills as well as audience evaluations and assessment.
- Teaching experience should be planned according to curriculum competencies appropriate to the stage in training.

Psychotherapy experience

- Give details of each area of psychotherapy experience in a standardised format that clearly communicates timescales, skills and techniques.
- Use the appropriate psychotherapy WPBAs.
- Use some method of linking your experience to reflective practice.

Management and leadership

- Provide a brief description of the experience, what skills were needed and what was learned.
- Bear in mind that experience and skills need to relate to competencies in the curriculum.

Reports, planning meetings and educational objectives

- There a number of reports that are required such as the induction meeting, personal development plan (PDP), mid-point review and educational supervisor's report.
- Use other records – such as records of supervision, on-call, PDPs – to further evidence competencies.
- There are a number of additional documents or achievements that can be valuable in the portfolio but remember that the curriculum is competency based, therefore explain anything you present. What exactly did you do? What are your skills? What feedback did you get?

Reference

General Medical Council (2013) *Ready for Revalidation: The Good Medical Practice Framework for Appraisal and Revalidation*. GMC.

CHAPTER 2

What is a portfolio?

What is a portfolio?

The concept of what a portfolio actually is has evolved over time (McMullan *et al*, 2003). Earlier definitions described the portfolio in more simple terms of a record of what someone has done (Redman, 1994). The definition has been extended to include giving regard to the dynamic process of learning, including a collection of different types of work that demonstrate achievement, learning and progress over time (Wenzel *et al*, 1998; Karlowicz, 2000). The portfolio can therefore be seen as a means of both assessment and recognition of learning (Knapp, 1975). Contemporary learning theory extends the portfolio's role as not only a document providing evidence of an individual's competence but also the record of professional development and how this has been achieved (Price, 1994). The developmental portfolio can therefore be seen as:

> 'A private collection of evidence, which demonstrates the continuing acquisition of skills, knowledge, attitudes, understanding and achievements. It is both retrospective and prospective, as well as reflecting the current stage of development and activity of the individual.' (Brown, 1995)

The portfolio should contain evidence from a number of sources chosen at the discretion of trainees, which should demonstrate particular competencies in different ways as well as recording personal reflections on the learning process and developmental needs. Put another way, the portfolio collects evidence by recording the process of development through experience, assessment and critical self-analysis or reflection.

The approach to the developmental portfolio

The theoretical approach to the developmental portfolio assumes that the individual is able to develop as an adult learner. As a part of this assumption trainees should (Knowles, 1975):

- be able to be self-directed

- have previous experience from which to learn
- be ready to learn, developing from experience
- be curious and motivated to develop.

Therefore, portfolio-based development is not passive learning facilitated and led by an expert but is informed by the process of reflecting on experience, so-called experiential learning. The dynamic interaction between theory, practice and experience is continuous and is demonstrated in Kolb's experiential learning cycle (Fig. 2.1).

In this way, Kolb's learning cycle is an attractive model for understanding the process of development as it explains the relationship between theory, such as concepts, and reflection on practice, such as experience and the testing of concepts. It is important to note that there is not a large body of empirical data to support this theoretical model (Quinn, 1998) and not all learning situations necessarily require the activation of all four stages of the cycle. An individual's motivation, interest and degree of innate curiosity will negatively or positively affect the degree to which the cycle is engaged.

The developmental portfolio is used increasingly in clinical training. The fact that the approach addresses the classic gap between theory and practice makes it desirable. There is evidence that portfolios can bring theory and practice closer together, as well as achieving subsequent improvements in practice and allowing the learner to take ownership of their development (Murrel *et al*, 1998) and gain a sense of responsibility (Wenzel *et al*, 1998). An additional benefit of this approach is that due to the continuous nature and structure of the portfolio, learners are encouraged to develop their skills in reflective practice, which then in turn enhances learning. However, this accountability, ownership and responsibility can be anxiety provoking. After a period in training, evidence of development will grow and confidence will increase, which should help to reduce such anxiety.

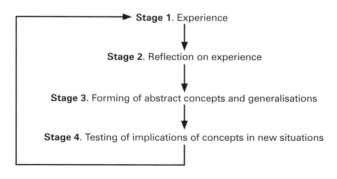

Fig. 2.1 Kolb's experiential learning cycle (Kolb, 1984).

Troubleshooting the portfolio

A recognised criticism of the portfolio is the time required to keep it up to date and acquiring sufficient evidence; indeed, trainees express anxiety about the nature and amount of evidence that should be collected (Mitchell, 1994). Such anxiety combined with the amount of time required negatively affects motivation (Mitchell, 1994). The best approach to counter this, which hopefully reduces anxiety, is integration and a change in learning culture. The portfolio is more useful as a learning tool if it is fully integrated into the training experience and always present, recording learning events, personal reflection and development plans as they occur. This may require trainees to timetable 'portfolio time' into their weekly plan and discuss the need for this with their supervisor in job planning. In this way the portfolio can be used to its potential and the workload needed for its upkeep is more evenly spread out. At the ARCP, the panel will be able to see that portfolios have been managed in this way and are more likely to result in a better outcome.

Too much information in the portfolio with numerous documents appended can be unwieldy and may only be meaningful to trainees, which may make the portfolios hard to interpret in the context of the ARCP and at other times of summative assessment. Equally, portfolios that have too little content may not effectively demonstrate the developmental process and thus become of limited value. It is impossible to be clear on 'how much is enough'. However, to be confident that sufficient evidence is gathered, the portfolio must be more than a collection or record of a range of work, experience and assessment, but must build on this by showing how the individual has reflected on these things, what has been learned and what still needs to be learned.

It is clear that reflective practice is key in adult learning and in the successful portfolio, where trainees identify gaps in their knowledge and competencies and take steps to address these needs. It is known that there can be a reluctance to engage in reflection on one's weaknesses and to some extent some see this process as intimidating and threatening (Snadden & Thomas, 1998). There is also uncertainty about how to reflect (Karlowicz, 2000) and some trainees may need guidance on this. For most trainees, reflection tends to occur through writing – writing ability varies between individuals (Snadden & Thomas, 1998) and there is a positive correlation between writing skills and positive reporting of the portfolio assessment by students (Mitchell, 1994). It is thought that, to a certain extent, the best way to overcome this is for trainees to focus on the developmental value of the portfolio, taking ownership of it and the process rather than seeing it as a tool for assessment. Hopefully, this approach will overcome the temptation not to fully disclose personal thoughts and feelings on experience. In this way the portfolio has a far greater developmental value and is more likely to be successful at the ARCP.

Learning theory suggests that the portfolio is a self-directed vehicle that promotes self-awareness, personal relfection, learning and accountability. For this to be possible the individual needs a degree of personal motivation and an adult learning style. The difficulty is that people have different learning styles (Snadden & Thomas, 1998) and therefore the developmental portfolio will not suit everybody. This difference in learning styles and the problem of some individuals finding the developmental portfolio approach difficult are to some extent unavoidable. However, one of the advantages of the developmental portfolio is that over time the use of this approach encourages and develops the very skills of self-relfection and personal development planning required for a successful portfolio.

The issue of ownership and self-direction is vital to the successful portfolio. Interestingly, it is known that trainees are less likely to engage with the portfolio if there is little or no pressure to be assessed (Harris *et al*, 2001). It is partly for this reason that the Royal College of Psychiatrists has concluded that there is a minimum number of WPBAs that should occur during a year in training (Bettison, 2010). These should occur throughout the year and not be left to the end, as it is impossible to use them to inform development if they do not address competence over time. The required minimum is exactly that; the more successful portfolios show that WPBAs occur in a range of situations, the number of which are related to trainees' developmental needs and should be fully integrated into reflective practice.

Educational theory

WPBA and competence

In assessing specialty training, one of the guiding principles is the recognition of the importance of reassuring the public about the safety and competence of doctors (Postgraduate Medical Education and Training Board, 2007). Workplace-based assessment provides a snapshot of what the doctor does in reality (i.e. it puts their performance into context), and it will therefore be conducted where trainees are currently working in the main (Postgraduate Medical Education and Training Board, 2007). So this is an assessment of trainees' actual performance as opposed to just their knowledge. Miller's pyramid helps to illustrate the progression from knowledge to competence as well as showing what level of performance common methods of assessment address in training (Fig. 2.2).

For a doctor to function competently, they need to acquire significant knowledge as well as a range of skills; these combine and contribute to competence. Therefore, as opposed to a known fact or skill, a specific competency may best be thought of as a constellation of abilities that include aspects of knowledge and skill as well as one's own experience and professional style. If portfolio evidence merely demonstrates the 'Knows' level of performance (e.g. a written examination result), it follows that it

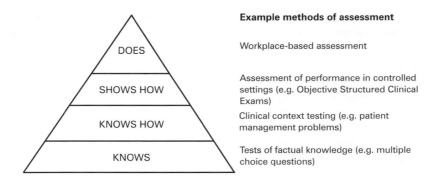

Example methods of assessment

Workplace-based assessment

Assessment of performance in controlled settings (e.g. Objective Structured Clinical Exams)

Clinical context testing (e.g. patient management problems)

Tests of factual knowledge (e.g. multiple choice questions)

Fig. 2.2 Miller's pyramid (Miller, 1990).

falls short of demonstrating the 'Does' level, i.e. competence. One of the reasons that there is an important distinction between other aspects of performance and competence is that a doctor's performance in controlled settings, such as examinations, is a poor predictor of performance in practice (Rethans *et al*, 2002).

Objective structured clinical methods of medical assessment are reproducible but often offer little scope for developmental feedback. Workplace-based assessment, on the other hand, has the capacity to provide such feedback that informs trainees' understanding of their developmental needs, which in turn drives the content of the portfolio. If competence was something distinct and relatively stable, then reproducible assessments could be designed specifically to assess competence. However, competence is specific to particular situations and does not necessarily generalise. It is for this reason that assessments and other evidence should sample widely across the curriculum and are made more meaningful by evidence of developmental feedback and the individual's own reflections. The portfolio must show that assessment and reflection inform learning.

The competency-based curriculum and triangulation

Criticisms of the competency-based curriculum include being simplistic and narrow (Talbot, 2002). Competencies, although holistic and covering a variety of attributes and skills, potentially become case or situation specific. Gathering sufficient supporting evidence of competencies by way of WPBAs and other forms of evidence from a broad range of assessors and contextual situations overcomes the problem of case specificity. In contrast to traditional approaches, where single methods of assessment were used (e.g. certified examinations), a range of sources of evidence are required in the portfolio.

Triangulation refers to how a particular competency can be evidenced and judged, to be attained using various sources of evidence. In this way over a training period, multiple assessors contribute to the portfolio evidence by using a variety of tools, as well as through judicious use of other forms of evidence. Information from one assessment can be compared with one or more forms of evidence relating to the same competency.

Bringing the evidence together – the portfolio

In medical training, the portfolio of competence can be defined as the 'dossier of evidence collected over a period in training that acts to demonstrate a doctor's education and skills in practice' (Wilkinson *et al*, 2002). Essentially, the portfolio shows the progression of trainees from novice to expert, driven by developmental assessment. The portfolio demonstrates competence in a number of ways:

- as a catalogue of WPBAs and other assessments
- as a developmental plan establishing developmental needs and how they have been addressed
- as a record of personal reflections regarding a wide range of clinical and non-clinical situations (these also inform development as well as being available to educational supervisors and the ARCP panel).

Interface with GMC revalidation

Revalidation started in 2012 and the GMC hopes to revalidate the majority of doctors by 2016. Revalidation of GMC-registered doctors is a single process with two potential outcomes: relicensing for all doctors and recertification for specialists.

Two key papers have driven the process forward: the White Paper *Trust, Assurance and Safety* (Hewitt, 2007) and *Medical Revalidation – Principles and Next Steps* (Department of Health, 2008). The principles forming the basis of the process include ensuring the safety and quality of care, sustaining confidence of the public, and identifying and addressing substandard practice. As such, doctors need to demonstrate that they are practising in accordance with the GMC's standards of good medical practice (General Medical Council, 2013) as well as standards appropriate to their specialty. These principles are strikingly similar to those set out by the GMC in their documents *The Trainee Doctor* (General Medical Council, 2011) and *Standards for Curricula and Assessment Systems* (General Medical Council, 2010).

The revalidation process will involve annual appraisal including formative and summative aspects, independent 360-degree feedback, resolution of any concerns, and positive affirmation of meeting of the standards of *Good Medical Practice* (General Medical Council, 2013) and those of the relevant college for specialists.

The annual appraisal will include the review of the portfolio presented by individual doctors, which is to be kept electronically in all likelihood. This is expected to bring together information from several sources, including: multisource feedback, continuing professional development (CPD), participation in audit, evaluation of clinical skills with CbD assessment, test of knowledge possibly using online CPD modules rather than examination, the use of clinical outcome measures, as well as learning from complaints and adverse incidents. This process is similar to the structure and types of evidence considered at the ARCP.

The call for revalidation and how consultants should manage a portfolio share a common history with the specialty trainee portfolio, including the use of multisource feedback, WPBA, reflective practice and professional development planning. For those already engaged in specialty training, revalidation will not be at all unfamiliar and indeed the majority of the evidence required for portfolios will already be routinely collected by trainees.

Key points to remember

- A successful portfolio is a developmental tool that builds a collection of evidence of experience, assessment of competence, self-reflection and personal development planning over time.
- Trainees should 'own' the portfolio by managing their own learning using the portfolio as a tool.
- The public want to be assured of the safety and professional competence of doctors.
- Portfolio evidence of competence must demonstrate performance in reality rather than the doctor's factual knowledge or abilities in controlled examinations.
- Evidence of achievement of competencies occurs by combining a variety of forms of evidence and assessments in various contexts and with multiple assessors.

Further reading

Royal College of Psychiatrists (2012) *Revalidation Guidance for Psychiatrists* (College Report CR172). Royal College of Psychiatrists.

References

Bettison S (2010) *WPBA Information*. Royal College of Psychiatrists (https://training.rcpsych.ac.uk/help/wpba-information).

Brown R (1995) *Portfolio Development and Profiling Nurses* (2nd edn). Quay Publications.

Department of Health (2008) *Medical Revalidation – Principles and Next Steps*. Department of Health.

General Medical Council (2010) *Standards for Curricula and Assessment Systems*. GMC.

General Medical Council (2011) *The Trainee Doctor: Foundation and Specialty, Including GP Training*. GMC.

General Medical Council (2013) *Good Medical Practice*. GMC.

Harris S, Dolan G, Fairbairn G (2001) Reflecting on the use of student portfolios. *Nurse Education Today*, **21**, 278–86.

Hewitt P (2007) *Trust, Assurance and Safety – The Regulation of Health Professionals in the 21st Century*. TSO (The Stationery Office).

Karlowicz KA (2000) The value of student portfolios to evaluate undergraduate nursing programs. *Nurse Educator*, **25**, 82–7.

Knapp J (1975) *A Guide for Assessing Prior Experience Through Portfolios*. Education Testing Service, Committee for the Assessment of Experiential Learning.

Knowles M (1975) *Self-Directed Learning: A Guide for Learners and Teachers*. Follet.

Kolb DA (1984) *Experiential Learning: Experience as the Source of Learning and Development*. Prentice Hall.

McMullan M, Endacott R, Gray MA, *et al* (2003) Portfolios and assessment of competence: a review of the literature. *Journal of Advanced Nursing*, **41**, 283–94.

Miller G (1990) The assessment of clinical skills/competence/performance. *Academic Medicine*, **65** (suppl), S63–7.

Mitchell M (1994) The views of students and teachers on the use of portfolios as a learning and assessment tool in midwifery education. *Nurse Education Today*, **14**, 38–43.

Murrel K, Harris L, Tomsett G, *et al* (1998) Using a portfolio to assess practice. *Professional Nurse*, **13**, 220–3.

Price A (1994) Midwifery portfolios: making reflective records. *Modern Midwife*, **4**, 35–8.

Postgraduate Medical Education and Training Board (2007) *Developing and Maintaining an Assessment System: A PMETB Guide to Good Practice*. PMETB.

Quinn FM (1998) *Continuing Professional Development in Nursing: A Guide for Practitioners and Educators*. Stanley Thomas.

Redman W (1994) *Portfolios for Development: A Guide for Trainers and Managers*. Kogan Page.

Rethans JJ, Norcini JJ, Barón-Maldonado M, *et al* (2002) The relationship between competence and performance: implications for assessing practice performance. *Medical Education*, **36**, 901–9.

Snadden D, Thomas ML (1998) Portfolios learning in general practice vocational training – does it work? *Medical Education*, **23**, 401–6.

Talbot M (2002) Monkey see, monkey do: a critique of the competency model in graduate medical education. *Medical Education*, **38**, 1–7.

Wenzel LS, Briggs KL, Puryear BL (1998) Portfolio: authentic assessment in the age of the curriculum revolution. *Journal of Nursing Education*, **37**, 208–12.

Wilkinson TJ, Challis M, Hobma SO, *et al* (2002) The use of portfolios for assessment of competence and performance of doctors in practice. *Medical Education*, **36**, 918–24.

CHAPTER 3

Lessons learned so far

The intention of this chapter is to capture the common questions and concerns raised by psychiatric trainees about portfolio-based learning in psychiatric training. Because of the often subtle answers to such questions, a structured, real question-and-answer format has been adopted. What follows is a transcript of a discussion about portfolio-based learning in psychiatric training, with Dr Samuel Dearman (S.D.) leading with questions from his position as a senior psychiatric trainee, Dr Damien Longson (D.L.) as an ARCP panel chair and Mrs Samantha Abbott (S.A.) as the head administrator of a medical education department. By reading this transcript, you should get a better understanding of why a portfolio is used, how to use it and how much to put in it, how the ARCP panel will judge your portfolio, as well as gaining improved understanding of the use of WPBAs, reflection, and meeting management and research competencies.

The developmental portfolio

S.D.: If we look at the portfolio itself as a place to start with, could you briefly describe what you think the portfolio needs to be from the position of the school of psychiatry, from an ARCP panel but also speaking as a trainer?

D.L.: It is a document owned by trainees, one of many they will have through their professional careers. What the panel really are trying to see is not whether trainees are developing habits that are going to become lifelong, but the way they learn, reflect and document things, and the way they drive their own personal development. It is a tool for the ARCP to use to make sure the individual develops properly. What the ARCP panel looks for is demonstration of that style of thinking. If there are serious deficiencies in terms of learning outcomes or things just have not been done at all, then clearly that's an issue and at the end of the day the curriculum requirements have to be met. We would be a lot more comfortable knowing that somebody is going to be a safe doctor for the next 20 or 30 years if their portfolio demonstrates the learning cycle. If the portfolio just demonstrates log book functions and no reflective processing, then we would be worried and would scrutinise more closely. But if overall it is a well-developed portfolio – well triangulated, well reflected – we will think, 'This is an adult learner, we are happy'.

S.D.: People might be familiar with keeping log books – the practice has been for many years to keep them – but what's the difference between keeping a log book and keeping a portfolio? And does a portfolio have any log book functions?

D.L.: There are log book functions, for example recording on-call activity, audit, supervision and teaching. The critical difference between the log book and the portfolio is that trainees need to demonstrate that they have thought about that experience, learned something new and plan more learning experiences so that they go round the loop. The portfolio is the loop element, a progressive demonstration of how you are going to be in the future, as well as how you have been in the past.

S.D.: I wonder about ownership and the need to understand the principles about how the portfolio is different. I wonder whether ownership is difficult for a lot of people; to have that sense of self-direction. Do you see that as an issue?

D.L.: Some trainees can see it as a tool to pass the ARCP and get their Certificate of Completion of Training (CCT). Persuading trainees that the portfolio is a lifelong learning tool is quite difficult. I think it's because at that stage of training many trainees do not realise, indeed we did not, that lifelong learning is part of the next 20–30 years of your life. It's like talking to consultants about developing portfolios for GMC revalidation – I think it's a shock for them as well.

S.A.: We try to address this at induction into training by doing a session on portfolios.

D.L.: I think the other thing that has changed is that now foundation trainees have portfolios and so we are finding that they are coming to us already with more of an understanding of portfolios. In fact, the ones coming through now have not really heard of log books.

S.D.: If we look at the model proposed for revalidation, which in many ways is quite similar to the model used for training in core and specialty levels now, the people who come through this system might actually be at an advantage because they are already working that way.

D.L.: Yes, I think that's the big change for existing consultants, because for them the learning curve is huge and I think for the average core trainee particularly, it's so much built into their everyday lives that it's much easier for them.

S.A.: We were discussing this recently and somebody was saying something about finishing training meaning 'No more ARCPs', so I said, 'I think it's called revalidation'.

S.D.: If we could steer back to some of the areas that cause anxiety among trainees looking at the portfolio. There are lots of different definitions about what a portfolio actually is, one of which is a private collection of evidence. I wonder who should have access to the portfolio and should some sections be restricted?

D.L.: We are all learning in that respect, and you are quite right in saying that early portfolios were very open documents and everybody had access to them. We are now realising that this does not work and there are a number of reasons why. One is that a trainee will be reluctant to put everything in if it demonstrates weakness and vulnerability or things that have not gone right, but we want them to put those in somehow because they are an important part of the cycle. I think the other aspect of that is that not everybody needs to see it anyway. I think we are coming to the conclusion, just like in National Health Service (NHS) appraisal, that there needs to be a locked and confidential section where trainees can put in something that is part of their internal world but that nobody else sees, unless they wanted them to.

The ARCP

S.D.: Something that often comes up is the question about how much is enough, what is sufficient evidence? The word triangulation suggests that a particular competency should be evidenced by at least three pieces of evidence. Is that entirely accurate?

D.L.: No. Triangulation does mean three but sometimes, again, I think it needs to demonstrate adult learning skills which are: 'How important is this competence?', 'How much have I demonstrated previously that I have achieved it?' and therefore, 'How much do I need to demonstrate that I have just refreshed it?' or 'Is it a brand new competence and do I need to demonstrate fairly robustly that I have actually acquired it?'. So it might be that you have demonstrated over years 1–3 that you have done very good risk assessments, you fully understand all the issues of self-harm, etc., and then in years 4–6 you don't need to demonstrate that you can manage self-harm assessments as competently. You need to demonstrate that you can still do it and you are still seeing patients who are at risk, i.e. you are involved with on-call and taking decisions but not necessarily having to triangulate that you can do self-harm assessments. You might just want to include a record of on-call that says you are doing them and you have had no serious untoward incidents, for example.

S.D.: But then, by logical extension a question arises: when the ARCP panel consider a year in training and trainees have taken the decision that they have done as described, developed their skills in that area and are now in a refreshing period if you will, how much consideration will the panel be able to give to previous x number of years, and how much will they refer directly to previous evidence?

D.L.: Well, the panel themselves will triangulate. So they will look at the training programme director's report that will say: 'I am satisfied that Dr Smith has previously met these competencies and there have been no issues in this current year in relation to that competence which gives me any cause for concern'. So that's evidence number one. Trainees will have written something in their portfolio to say, for example, intended learning objective (ILO) related to risk assessments – this competence was largely achieved in years 1–3, however, this year I have maintained it in the following kind of ways, and the panel can access previous portfolios.

S.D.: I wonder how well people appreciate that. It might be a message that I think trainees need to hear more.

D.L.: The classic one really is probity, which I know is one of the hardest things to demonstrate, but the GMC says that as doctors we must demonstrate our probity at every stage of our career. So just because we have achieved the competence of knowing what probity is, you have then got to demonstrate ongoing probity in practice for the rest of your career. The GMC have said that for trainees it is the same process as their learning portfolio, so you can't ignore all these things just because you have learned them previously – you still have to do them.

S.D.: What about time? Trainees often give feedback saying there is just not enough time to complete the portfolio and to do the work which they are contracted to do, and to perhaps have a life on top of that.

D.L.: Yes. Consultants say exactly the same, that there is so much work required for revalidation. It is partly about using your portfolio consistently throughout the year, and partly about using it smartly, so that it helps you identify the areas on which you need to focus your learning and clinical experiences.

S.A.: It is difficult. The ARCP can fall right in the middle of an exam, but the rules are you have to have an ARCP looking at your portfolio and the competencies have to be met. I guess it's about planning your year. Workplace-based assessments have to be spread over a period. Realistically, if trainees do it properly and go to do their WPBA knowing which competency they meet, then it needn't all be left to the end.

D.L.: I think there is a reality for employers: it takes a lot of time and it has to be factored into job plans. This is part of the modern NHS.

Similarly, having time for teaching and training is not opted into job plans and medical students are not included in job plans, yet it is all part of the new economy and I think that the trusts are lagging behind the regulations in some respects.

S.A.: That's just the reality in which trainees train. So, can you give me a sense of what the practical solutions might be?

D.L.: I think for trainees, it is negotiating with their trainers that they need some time set aside, that part of their supervision is discussing their portfolio and being reminded to do their portfolio, and so on, so that it is an active part of trainees' working life, as opposed to something that has to be done extra to it.

S.A.: If it is incorporated into their supervision and everyday working life – like we said, it should be an educational tool – then it is not going to be something that is left to the end of the year and rushed to be put together. It should be ongoing with your supervisor, so basically the work is done.

S.D.: It might be helpful to get a sense of how the ARCP process actually runs. I suppose I am thinking about, given that the panel can only consider the evidence before it, how much time of scrutiny will each portfolio get altogether.

D.L.: It depends on the quality of the portfolio, how well constructed the evidence is and whether there have been previous problems or not. So, for example, trainee A who has previously had outcome 1's, who then presents a very well-triangulated portfolio where all the sections have been completed and there are no obvious major gaps, we will occasionally spot check that evidence for a competence is genuine evidence for a competence. This will result in a lower-level scrutiny than in trainee B who has previously had outcome 2's and 3's, who has been struggling and has had gaps in their portfolio. For trainee B we will check that a WPBA actually evidences competency in the area of the curriculum the trainee claims it does. For example, if a trainee has uploaded a document under 'audit', which simply states they have not done the audit yet, this would result in a higher level of scrutiny of their entire portfolio. In case you think that's not fair, every other quality control process in the NHS is like that now. It's light touch unless light touch is not appropriate. So, a straightforward ARCP takes 15–30 minutes to review the evidence and another 15–30 minutes to discuss.

S.A.: I think you also have to look at the process that has happened before it actually gets to panel. We have the training programme director reviews twice a year, so we already know whether there are any problems. And then prior to the ARCP we go through the portfolio and document that everything that should be there is there – that all the competencies do have a link – and then the half hour is for the panel member to discuss the quality of the evidence rather than the amount.

S.D.: Following on from that, having run a few rounds of ARCPs now, I wonder whether there are repeated 'heart sink' moments, repeated mistakes that occur that you pick up on.

D.L.: I'm sure Sam will have even more examples than I have. The most common is just failing to submit mandatory evidence.

S.D.: For example?

D.L.: GMC survey, school survey, evidence of attending induction or breakaway – all those kinds of things that are statutory and we know trainees have done them and they are just not submitting the evidence, and that is just lack of attention to detail really.

S.A.: I think they are simply not including things. The biggest problem is that they might be competent but they just have not included the piece of evidence that demonstrates this. It might be referred to in the training programme director's report or the educational supervisor's report or even by the trainee, but it is not physically there.

D.L.: A common one is audit. To say I've done an audit or to have the title of the audit does not demonstrate competence. In the same way, if you attend a course it does not mean you are competent at it. Within your audit evidence you must show not only that have you done the audit but that you understand the principles for it and why it is important.

S.D.: So, for example, it might be helpful for them to link that to reflective practice or to get some feedback from others about the process and the application of it, is that right?

D.L.: Absolutely. Because a medical student or an administrative worker could do an audit. The practicalities of doing an audit are quite straightforward. The real competence is understanding why you are doing it in the first place and why it is relevant to your professional practice.

S.D.: I wonder whether some trainees find frustrating the perception that the portfolio and the ARCP process are not designed to recognise particular achievement or even excellence. Is that accurate?

D.L.: Yes, we recognise that we all struggle with that. Using the portfolio to demonstrate excellence is not in the Gold Guide.[1] The ARCP is about competence. I think that to say you can do something competently better than somebody else would worry patients.

S.A.: The very good trainees are easy to spot by their portfolios – they are easy to understand and you can see clearly why those pieces of evidence match that competency. On the other hand, in a struggling trainee who has really fought to put the evidence in there, you can't actually always tell how that piece of evidence fits that competency.

---

1. *A Reference Guide for Postgraduate Specialty Training in the UK ('The Gold Guide 2010')*. Health Education England, 2010.

D.L.: But it's how you reward that excellence and it may be that the portfolio is not the right tool. In my experience, when interviewing people for jobs, trainees who have very good portfolios and confidently discuss them actually tend to get the better jobs.

S.D.: A basic question perhaps: I understand that ARCP panels hate plastic pockets when using paper portfolios which are otherwise commonly used to protect paper documents. Is that true? And if so, why?

S.A.: It is true, but it's only a problem where trainees stick a whole pack of documents into one wallet, whereas if they put them back to back you can flick over the pages more easily. I guess, how they do that – shoving it all in one polly pocket – says a lot about them as a person and their organisation skills.

D.L.: There is no reason why they can't use a four-hole punch, for example, and dividers. The dividers have the same purpose as individual polly pockets but at least they make the portfolio browsable.

Being called to the ARCP panel

S.D.: The minority of trainees will be called before the ARCP panel, but I suspect there is still an air of mystery about that. I wonder whether you can give a sense of what it is like? I suppose specifically about how formal it is, how critical it is and is it stressful?

D.L.: From a trainee's perspective it is extremely stressful and that's acknowledged. The external reviewers and the lay reviewers who come to our panels and comment on the process say that it is a very supportive, very emphatic, very careful process, but we do know that from trainees' perspectives it certainly does not feel like that at all. It is absolutely not meant to be punitive, it is there to be supportive and give trainees an opportunity to present their evidence. I think that one thing that trainees misunderstand is that just because they have come to panel B[2] does not necessarily mean there are educational issues; it means there are things that need clarifying, and in some cases trainees come along, clarify the evidence, say 'I forgot to submit it, and here's the evidence' and that's the end of the process. But trainees say that being called to panel B is a slur on their education forever; it is not. I know there are a lot of people there; we have a list of statutory people as required by the Gold Guide – it feels like a room full. A large proportion of the remainder come up for an outcome 2, and that's often for relatively minor

2. This is the name of the panel in the North Western Deanery which trainees will attend to look in more detail at their portfolio if it is felt there is a reason that the portfolio cannot be given an outcome 1 (i.e. pass) after the first review.

things. That's what outcome 2 is – it's not a concern about trainees, it's simply that there were competencies not demonstrated. And then a very small proportion of trainees come for an outcome 3, and those trainees know that they have more enduring difficulties.

Workplace-based assessment

S.D.:   At this time, there is a set minimum required for the number of each type of WPBA per period of training. I wonder what your reaction is to that, and whether the recommendation of the minimum number to be done can be misinterpreted by trainees?

S.A.:   I think 'minimum number' is misleading.

D.L.:   It is educationally misleading. I suppose the numbers have been set in a way that if you do fewer than that, it is inconceivable that you demonstrate the principles of adult learning. If a trainee presents just the minimum number of assessments, the panel is going to be more concerned about their portfolio and they will scrutinise it more thoroughly and spend longer on it. Whereas if there are lots of WPBAs there and they are well described and used as evidence, the panel is going to feel that this trainee understands that these are formative things that are driving their education and they are engaged in their training.

S.D.:   Yes, the concept of engagement in training: how does that marry up with simply meeting the minimum requirements? I think that is the difficulty.

S.A.:   You just would not be able to get through. You would not be able to meet all your competencies with the current minimum.

S.D.:   Do you know that for a fact?

S.A.:   Yes, if you use two ACEs you would have to use those ACEs to cover every single item in the curriculum.

D.L.:   I think you need to be careful of that because the evidence for a competence is not just a WPBA. Trainees could do it by having lots of other evidence, but usually they are the weaker portfolios where there are a number of other issues. The Royal College of Psychiatrists has produced guidance on the kinds of ACEs that you need to do and the mini-ACEs for all the ILOs. There are basically 19 different ACEs with 19 different ILOs for each year of training, so that is not consistent with the minimum number of 2 or 4, etc. So, I think if a trainee looks at all their ILOs, they can't but do many more than the bare minimum.

S.D.:   I wonder whether you could spell out clearly, how a WPBA can be used in benchmarking at the beginning of a period in training.

D.L.: The College is now going to require trainees to do a WPBA (an ACE) within the first month of their job, and that it goes into their portfolio and then for the rest of that 6-month job, the portfolio is partly built around that initial ACE, which will set the benchmark for what needs to be learned that year. So if it is set around that initial ACE and the initial PDP, then you could see how the portfolio becomes integral to that trainee's work experience for the next 6–12 months.

S.D.: That leads me on to my next question about balance. I wonder what the balance should be between pre-booked, timetabled WPBA and more spontaneous WPBA?

D.L.: I think that the question splits theory and practice. In theory, I would say they should all be spontaneous WPBAs. They were born in the acute surgical specialties – someone would turn up in accident and emergency with a particular pathology, trainees would grab their educational supervisor and say 'Have a look at me examining this patient'. I think that is ideally how it should be for us as well. I know that in practice the consultants aren't always available, it's difficult to get the assessment completed and that WPBAs get pre-booked because trainees say to consultants, 'Can you clear your clinic a week on Thursday so that when I do my clinic you can supervise me?', and so on. I think that is a pragmatic balance. Consultants pre-booking patients for trainees to do WPBAs on a specific thing is completely the wrong way round – that certainly should not happen.

S.D.: I wonder whether one approach to planning WPBAs is to map out areas of the curriculum competencies with possible WPBAs?

D.L.: The right way to plan your WPBAs is to look at what competencies you need to demonstrate. Think to yourself, 'How could I demonstrate that competence?' and you might say, 'That might be with a workplace-based assessment'. It might be with a whole variety of other things, but if you do WPBA, it must be driven by a need to demonstrate competence, not the other way round. So when you ask your consultant or trainer to do an assessment with you, you say to them 'I need to demonstrate ILOs 1, 7 and 14'.

S.A.: Trainees should take along a_copy of the curriculum showing the knowledge, skills and attitudes required for each ILO to their WPBA. The best trainees will say 'OK, it's ILO 1 and it was clinical history', because if you just put ILO 1, you've got quite a few things in there, haven't you? So, it is about getting consultants, or whoever is assessing you, to think about what aspect of ILO 1 they are looking at and actually judge that aspect specifically.

D.L.: So, this means using the curriculum to drive the assessment. The ARCP panel needs to make sure that there is evidence of having met the curriculum and the curriculum is defined by the competencies, so the competencies and the curriculum drive the whole process.

Reflective practice

S.D.: I think that reflective practice is a particularly challenging area and for some trainees it can be a problem, partly because we know it relates to particular kinds of writing skills. I think it has also got something to do with the perception of weakness or attracting criticism. We have touched on it to some extent already, but how do you think reflective practice fits into the portfolio and, specifically, how important is it to the ARCP?

D.L.: We need to know two things about an educational experience. We often need trainees to describe the actual experience itself, particularly if it was a WPBA. We need them to say, 'This is what I did, these were the clinical issues that arose, these are the competencies that I intend to demonstrate'. A factual objective account and followed by a reflective element. What the panel will want to see is that they document and present sufficient reflection to show they understand the principles, why reflection is important, and I think that to demonstrate vulnerability is a strength. If you go around thinking that nothing is your fault and that you are always right and that your reflection is that everyone else is letting you down, then you will be a very dangerous doctor. It is actually saying that 'This nearly happened and gosh that was awful'. Sometimes reflecting on the incidents of others as well – 'There but for the grace of God, go I'. Those are all very useful things that demonstrate conscious awareness of the risks, and the panel does not always want to see exact detail of the reflection, they want to see that the person is reflecting thoughtfully.

S.A.: Trainers and trainees need training on what reflection is there for. I think it is true that sometimes you do get a trainer who will see somebody who has reflected a lot and see it as a weakness, but I'm sure that weakness would show up elsewhere and in the WPBAs if that was the case.

S.D.: I suppose it's not only the fact of it, but what you do with the awareness of areas you need to improve on and how you demonstrate that you have improved.

D.L.: I think that if you can be intellectually honest, there is virtually nothing that you do where you can't go away and think, 'What could I have done differently?' Clinical interaction is not perfect, it is perhaps 95% perfect and what do you do with that 5%? You go away and think about it and it's capturing that really and striving to improve.

S.D.: Which then leads to the following question: do you think that trainees evidence reflective practice well? If not, what advice would you give for it to be improved?

D.L.: There is a wide range. The very poor ones are totally concrete, which is 'This is what I did'. The ones that are worrying are both concrete and self-explanatory: 'This is what I did, everybody else let me down but luckily I was right in the end', through to profoundly reflective, insightful records. So, what can we do about it? We have been running some training for consultants, as everybody knows that doctors are not very good at it. This is a genuinely complex skill that people need to be trained in, and it's not something that you necessarily do intuitively.

S.A.:   Some trainees worry that reflection shows weakness or will reveal imperfections. There is another side to the coin as well – it also shows some trainees who reflect but beat themselves up about things when they are actually doing fantastically.

Research skills and management experience

S.D.:   A specific anxiety in the portfolio and competency-based curriculum in psychiatry, arguably more than in other specialties, is research. Core trainees are often anxious about whole projects being required. Does the ARCP panel expect a whole project, specifically from core trainees or even higher trainees?

D.L.:   No. If you look at the guidance, for example the old age specialty curriculum, it mentions research in very general terms. It is acknowledged that some trainees are going to be career academics, whereas others have very limited interest in research and just need to demonstrate an understanding of the basic principles, and the importance of research and how it fits into day-to-day clinical practice. All the panels know this – we have never struggled with it. Trainees bring it up all the time, but the panels feel quite comfortable that the training programme director will say trainees are not heading in a research direction but they are quite competent, they have done a couple of small things and it's fine. So, we are quite relaxed about it.

S.D.:   I think that's probably quite encouraging to trainees. I wonder whether there are similar anxieties or uncertainties about management experience?

D.L.:   I think, realistically, every consultant has to be a manager. If you look at the competencies, there is one for the doctor as a manager but there isn't one as a researcher. We can avoid the management competencies. Trainees need to be trained sufficiently so that when they do become young consultants, they have enough confidence to be able to start their management roles. They don't have to be competent managers at this stage, they just have to be able to get the ball rolling. I think it is different to research. Research is a very specific skill for a few individuals.

S.A.:   I think some trainees have difficulty filling that box because they don't actually know the management that they are doing. A year 1 core trainee (CT1) never realises that they are demonstrating skills in management, but they are actually doing quite a lot.

S.D.: An example?

S.A.: Well, they might be on a ward round or managing a patient; OK, it is under supervision but they are still undertaking management roles in there, aren't they?

D.L.: Yes, I think that's right, because managing a patient involves negotiating with the family, negotiating with ward staff; there is a whole range of negotiation skills, planning skills and timekeeping skills. So, that is management. If you look at something that a second- or third-year trainee might do, like running the rota, I mean that is really becoming quite complex management. Although it is a simple task, you have got to pacify your colleagues, keep the surface safe, negotiate swops, tensions and arguments. That's quite advanced management and yet very few trainees put those down as management experience, because they see management as being 'that kind of formal thing' that you do in trust headquarters.

S.A.: It is similar to trainees who say they have been on some management course but they cannot put that into practice. The question is how does that change your everyday practice.

D.L.: It's not only that management is a political process, which is something that happens on trust boards and in trust buildings, it is a competence which involves working with people, managing relationships and so on, and that is the competence we are trying to find, not whether you can run a trust.

A take-home message

S.D.: Just finally, if I pushed you to give one sentence of advice on managing a portfolio successfully from your perspective, what would it be?

D.L.: Leave no gaps.

S.A.: Do not leave it to the end of the year.

ˍanising the portfolio

The portfolio is potentially a huge file of reports, assessments, documents and projects that one can very easily get lost in. If this mound of material is not understandable or easy to read, this is a difficulty not only for trainees but also for the ARCP panel. That is not to say that ARCP panels cannot be bothered with disorganised portfolios but simply that disorganisation significantly increases the risk of information being missed. The portfolio needs divisions and a table of contents, and each section can be tabbed to make reading easier. An indexing system should complement the basic structure of the portfolio; this references the various sources of evidence relating to specific competencies. A suggested structure for a table of contents is given in Box 4.1. Notice that this is kept very simple and it is immediately obvious as to the nature of the divisions.

Box 4.1 Example of a portfolio table of contents

1 Summary of posts
2 Summary of evidence/index
3 Appraisal reports
4 Workplace-based assessments
5 Psychotherapy experience
6 Audit and research experience
7 Professional development planning and reviews
8 Leadership and management experience
9 Teaching
10 Training and courses
11 Other relevant experience and documentation
12 Record of educational supervision
13 Record of on-call activity
14 Special interest reports (higher trainees)

The importance of indexing in demonstrating triangulated evidence

It is perhaps not immediately obvious to all trainees that an index can serve as a vital part of a successful portfolio. Many online or e-portfolios have an indexing system built into them, but if not, or you are using a paper-based portfolio, consider the need for a good system that identifies the location of evidence during the ARCP, as the ARCP is ultimately the submission of evidence. At the ARCP the panel can only consider the evidence they have before them, i.e. the contents of the portfolio. This single folder needs to communicate development during a year in training. The panel review in excess of 50 portfolios at each sitting. Imagine the difficulty for the panel when a portfolio whether full of documents, paper or electronic, are put before them claiming to demonstrate professional competence over a broad range of areas but does not tell them where to find the piece of work they need to see. One can quite easily understand how after seeing 20 poorly organised portfolios the already weighty process could accidentally overlook evidence. It is not dissimilar to the experience of clinical examinations and good exam technique. For example, a student would lose marks in an Objective Structured Clinical Examination if they neglected to introduce themselves, clearly explain the task at hand and what they will be doing. This would be an example of poor communication skills. Portfolios that fail to clearly communicate their content risk evidence being overlooked and not demonstrating work that may in fact be of excellent quality. The main motivator here should be not to sell yourself short simply because the portfolio is hard to read.

What a good index, or summary of evidence, does

In the future, the curriculum is sure to change but the principal need for organisation will stand. There are key points in creating an understandable index and these should answer the following questions.

- Is the index easy to read?
- Is it obvious where to find the evidence/work?
- Is there a clear description of the competency?
- Is it clear that there are multiple sources of evidence for each competency? Has it been triangulated?

When one reads the index of evidence, it is clear that there is triangulated and sufficient evidence (see Chapter 2, p. 8 for a discussion of the educational theory regarding triangulation). For example, a single WPBA relating to an emergency assessment does not completely evidence competency in this area, but if this is triangulated with attendance at risk management training with personal reflections and an audit regarding local adherence to trust risk assessment policy, this significantly expands on this competency. An indexing system makes clear that evidence is triangulated and where it is located within the portfolio.

In the following paragraphs two examples of indexing, one poor and one good, are considered. These examples are hypothetical and serve only to illustrate the points discussed earlier.

A poor indexing system

Competency	Evidence
Medical Expert: ILO 7	Case-based discussion – workplace-based assessments

In this example, although this is readable it is not meaningful or sufficiently informative. The following questions arise: 'What aspect of competence is ILO 7 – is it prioritising information in emergencies or is it something else?', 'Is the evidence presented as achievement of that competency?', 'Where are the WPBAs?', 'Is it all the CbDs or specific ones?' and 'Is this the only evidence for this competency?' Clearly, there is room for improvement here. Contrast this with the better example below.

A good indexing system

Aspects	Competency	Evidence of achievement	
Medical Expert: ILO 7	Management of severe and enduring mental illness	Section 4.	Evidence of competence statement, Dr Brown, consultant supervisor
		Section 6.	WPBA mini-Peer Assessment Tool, Rounds 1 and 2
		Section 6.	WPBA ACE Nos. 2 and 4
		Section 6.	WPBA mini-ACE No. 2
		Section 6.	WPBA CbD Nos. 1–3
		Section 10.	Audit and research. Does completion of electronic care programme approach documents comply with policy requirements on the assessment of health and social needs?

In this example it is clear to the reader that the evidence relates to a particular competency under a more general aspect of the curriculum. The triangulated evidence is presented and achievement is stated. Within the evidence column, it is clear that the trainee is presenting various pieces of work and assessments relating to this competency. It is clear exactly where in the portfolio evidence is found and it helps to reference exactly which WPBA is relevant. An additional tip would be to add a further column, which the educational supervisor can sign as an endorsement.

Presenting a single example of evidence is insufficient. Time should be taken when assessments have been completed to ensure that the developmental and evidential potential has been maximised; that is, the curriculum should be read closely, as each assessment can track on to aspects of various competencies (Chapter 7 expands on this). However, and quite obviously, the more salient the work done, the more valuable the portfolio will be.

Key points to remember

- Organisation and reference to clearly indexed, triangulated evidence at the start of the portfolio sets the tone.
- Make it user-friendly; clearly state the competency and give clear, specific locations of evidence.

CHAPTER 5

Managing your workplace-based assessments

Workplace-based assessments have become a common formative assessment tool in all areas of postgraduate medical education. There is no pass/fail, so WPBAs should provide feedback to trainees about developing skills required to carry out their work competently. Workplace-based assessments may also highlight areas that require more attention and so can inform future PDPs. They have become an important part of postgraduate medical training as they are considered to demonstrate effective and frequent review and appraisal of trainee doctors. They test an individual's skills, knowledge and behaviour against GMC-approved curricula (General Medical Council, 2010) in a wide variety of clinical contexts and allow trainees to demonstrate progress in their skills in their workplace. Workplace-based assessments also have the opportunity to identify trainees who are struggling, as mandatory WPBAs oblige closer supervision than would otherwise exist without them. Assessment of competence in this way can be argued to be an obligation of professionalism and professional duty, given that the public has expressed a desire for improvements in self-regulation (Cruess & Cruess, 2006).

Workplace-based assessments have their limitations too, such as not being reliable as the only source of assessment for trainees and being completed to 'get the numbers', rather than using a WPBA as a valuable educational experience for which it is intended. Many WPBAs require assessors to rate trainees on a number of different scales. Low scores can leave trainees feeling like they have failed, despite the formative nature of WPBAs. Senior clinical staff and educational supervisors can often struggle to find the time to complete WPBAs, so a supervisor must be prepared to make time to observe and provide feedback. Finally, standardising judgement can be difficult (General Medical Council, 2010) and so WPBAs may not be as reliable as summative assessments.

The WPBA is one of the cornerstones of assessment structure. The requirements in terms of numbers per training post are actually relatively small when one takes time to reflect on the number of competencies a trainee is expected to demonstrate each year. When used well the WPBA is very helpful and can cover a wide range of competencies. Workplace-based assessments cover a variety of skills and information, and the upshot of this is that they convey a great deal about a trainee's skills. This information therefore needs to be managed and well presented within the portfolio. Like the indexing of evidence discussed in Chapter 4, an online portfolio may already have a system in place to manage and present WPBAs.

How WPBA is recorded varies across deaneries. Some use paper forms and others electronic. For certain types of WPBA, such as the mini-Peer Assessment Tool (mini-PAT) or patient feedback, a number of individuals complete a 'round' of assessments which can then be summarised and compared against the trainee's self-appraisal. Whatever system is used, the principles and guidance in this chapter should apply.

Before a WPBA is conducted, it is good practice to refer to the curriculum and look at the various aspects of each ILO so that the feedback can relate directly to the curriculum. Within the curriculum for each year in training, the Royal College of Psychiatrists has suggested particular WPBAs for particular patients and clinical situations for each ILO. This underlines the need for familiarity with the curriculum as soon as training begins, using it to produce developmentally useful WPBAs.

Being orderly

First, it seems logical to present each type of WPBA together; that is, order all ACEs one after the other in chronological order, then mini-ACEs, etc. It may make sense to provide a cover page for WPBAs; this could number each WPBA, with a brief title and a sentence explaining the situation. Underneath this title you could also choose to state the related competencies. This brings order to a lot of information and makes immediately clear the relevance of each WPBA. Box 5.1 shows an example of what such a cover page might look like.

Making the most of every WPBA

The ability to reflect is considered central to competence. The better-developed portfolios make WPBAs even more useful and informative by linking them to a further document that provides the following:

- additional text briefly clarifying the context of the assessment, any salient clinical issues and ILOs, and why the assessment was undertaken (e.g. why, where, who); it seems sensible to utilise reflective practice documents, but a document covering the above aspects is probably just as good
- a statement of personal reflections of the experience, including any observations and feedback received; this might include positive aspects such as skills that should be capitalised on in future practice

---

Box 5.1 Example of a WPBA cover page

Workplace-based assessment: case-based discussion

CbD 1: Applying for leave for a restricted patient with a changeable mental state

Related competencies include: mental state examination, tailored management, knowledge and application of legislation (Mental Health Act 1983), detention, decision-making, following code of practice, good practice in risk management, liaison with other services (e.g. Ministry of Justice)

CbD 2: Regarding the management of agitated depression in a physically disabled older adult

Related competencies include: prioritising information, mental state and physical examination, diagnosis, correspondence, change in functioning, tailored care planning, decision matrix regarding level of risk, physical incapacity and ethics, liaison with other services (secure rehabilitation and physicians)

CbD 3: Risk assessment and an acute stress reaction

Related competencies include: prioritising information, mental state examination, diagnosis, correspondence, change in functioning, tailored care planning including supportive psychotherapy, good practice regarding risk management, liaison with other services

---

- some kind of action or plan that informs your continuing professional development.

An example of a well-presented mini-ACE linked to reflective practice and professional development is shown in Box 5.2.

Developing WPBAs

Current WPBAs available are ACE, mini-ACE and CbD. These may not be adequate for the competency being assessed. The North Western Deanery has developed a WPBA called the Direct Observation of Non-Clinical Skills (DONCS). This allows for feedback in domains such as teaching, chairing meetings, writing reports, etc. With a DONCS, trainees are assessed on the seven areas of competency required by doctors identified by CanMEDS (Frank, 2005), which has been adopted by the Royal College of Psychiatrists for the development of the curriculum (e.g. Royal College of Psychiatrists, 2010). These seven areas are: medical expert, communicator, collaborator, manager, health advocate, scholar and professional. Direct Observation of Non-Clinical Skills is currently just being used for higher trainees, so the marks for each of the areas are as follows:

- significantly short of readiness for consultant practice
- approaching readiness for consultant practice
- ready for consultant practice
- unable to comment.

Box 5.2 Example of a mini-Assessed Clinical Encounter (mini-ACE)

Setting: Crisis/emergency   Diagnosis 1: F20.9
Previous contact: 0   Complexity: Moderate

	Below expectations	Satisfactory	Better than expected
1 History taking			✓
2 Mental state examination	✓		
3 Communication skills		✓	
4 Clinical judgement	✓		
5 Professionalism		✓	
6 Organisation/efficiency		✓	
7 Overall clinical care	✓		
8 Based on this assessment, how would you rate the trainee's performance at this stage of training?	✓		

Anything particularly good?
Good use of conversational style and opening questioning.

Any areas for development?
To incorporate legal framework regarding decision-making capacity into clinical assessment.

Agreed action
• To look at the Mental Capacity Act 2005 Code of Practice, especially Chapter 4.
• Consider the need for further training regarding Mental Capacity Act course.
• Plan to observe a capacity assessment.

Reflective note: self-appraisal of learning

Brief description of learning of this experience
I was assessed, with a mini-ACE, interviewing a patient with acute psychosis who was no longer taking their antipsychotic medication. They had presented in crisis. I was assessing their understanding of their mental health and potential risks, ILOs 2 and 3.

What did you learn?
Although I felt able to manage the interview with respect to levels of arousal and engagement, there was room for improvement with my assessment of his ability to consent to treatment, including how I incorporate the Mental Capacity Act into my assessments.

What feedback did you get from your assessor?
To sit in on a capacity assessment as well as seeking further training in the Mental Capacity Act (formal or informal).

In light of this experience, what do you need to learn about, and how will you adapt your PDP?
I will refer myself to the Mental Capacity Act Code of Practice and undertake the recommended e-learning course, and discuss this in educational supervision. I will also observe my consultant as well as another member of the team performing a capacity assessment to look at different approaches. I will plan another mini-ACE to include 'capacity' within 6 weeks.

These marks will likely have more meaning for trainees rather than the numerical score of 1–6 on other WPBAs. A DONCS for core trainees could also be used, but 'higher specialist training' could be used in place of 'consultant practice'.

Key points to remember

- Present WPBAs in a logical sequence and consider a covering page.
- Make it clear what the WPBA was about and link it to reflective practice and your professional development.

References

Cruess RL, Cruess SR (2006) Teaching professionalism: general principles. *Medical Teacher*, **28**, 205–8.

Frank JR (ed.) (2005) *The CanMEDS 2005 Physician Competency Framework: Better Standards. Better Physicians. Better Care.* The Royal College of Physicians and Surgeons of Canada.

General Medical Council (2010) *Workplace-Based Assessment: A Guide for Implementation.* GMC.

Royal College of Psychiatrists (2010) *A Competency Based Curriculum for Specialist Core Training in Psychiatry: Core Training in Psychiatry CT1-CT3.* Royal College of Psychiatrists.

CHAPTER 6

Reflective practice and self-appraisal of learning

Central to personal development and demonstrating one's ability to learn from experience is the ability to reflect. Reflective practice or self-appraisal of learning notes present a standardised method of recording experience and personal reflections of what was learned and how this might inform personal development.

How to record reflective practice

Much like other parts of the portfolio, the recording and presenting of reflective practice should follow a standardised format that presents a summary of each aspect of reflective practice. Trainees and the ARCP panel need to understand the experience, learning and reference to any developmental needs. The actual form used is not important but trainees should ensure they record the following:

- a brief description of the experience, assessment or learning situation
- any feedback received (e.g. from a supervisor, a patient, a colleague)
- a summary of personal reflections – what was learned, what went well, what could have gone better as well as the emotional impact of the situation
- a note of any actions needed to take as a result of feedback and/or reflection (i.e. professional development).

It should be remembered that reflection or self-appraisal happens, or should happen, all the time and in many different contexts. Therefore, trainees should ensure they record reflective practice across a broad range of clinical and non-clinical domains. Examples include: ethical dilemmas, times when another team member dealt with a difficult situation well, when personal decision-making could have been better, when and why it was felt that a good protocol was vital in clinical audit, etc. An example of a reflective note completed in an informative and useful way is provided later in the chapter.

The difficult question of where to file reflective notes

Broadly speaking, trainees have three choices as to which section of the portfolio to file reflective notes in.

Method 1: A separate section titled 'reflective practice'

Filing reflective notes in a dedicated section will result in a number of forms recording thoughts concerning a variety of experiences and learning situations. The key therefore would be to make this section orderly and logical so that the information does not become unmanageable, missed and even uninteresting. To avoid this pitfall, the section could begin with its own contents page, which categorises learning experiences in a logical way. This would enable the reader to quickly understand the broad range of clinical, managerial and academic aspects of psychiatry that trainees reflect on and learn from as a matter of their practice. A contents page of this type might look something like that shown in Box 6.1.

The downside of applying this method is that although this is undoubtedly a well-ordered approach, it may still be lengthy and require some effort to read and be used to develop from. A further question to consider is salience – for example, is a reflective note concerning a WPBA more informative if it is filed immediately after that assessment? Method 2 considers this question.

Box 6.1 Contents page for reflective practice

Section 4. Reflective practice
Summary of reflective notes

On-call work and emergencies	No. 1–6
Ethical dilemmas	No. 7–9
Interview skills	No. 10–14
Relationships with colleagues	No. 15–20
Leadership experience	No. 21–22
Working as a teacher	No. 23–26
Giving evidence	No. 27–29
Applying research evidence to clinical practice	No. 30–31
Workplace-based assessments	No. 32–39

Method 2: Filing reflective notes where they are most relevant

There is a good argument to say that reflective notes are more informative if they follow the information they are relevant to, such as a WPBA. Clearly, a reflective note that is completed in sufficient detail following a WPBA readily demonstrates reflective practice and means that trainees and those reading the portfolio do not have to refer to other parts of the document.

In this way, reflective notes can potentially be filed with WPBAs, other formal assessments, audit and research, management experience, etc. Seemingly, therefore, a separate section for reflective practice is unnecessary. However, what about those experiences that do not clearly fit into other sections but have good learning value and important reflective aspects? Consider method 3 below.

Method 3: Using what works – a flexible filing system

There are merits and downsides of both a dedicated reflective practice section and filing specific notes where relevant. For some trainees adopting both of these methods is probably the best solution. This might mean that reflective notes linked to WPBAs are filed in the WPBA section, and reflections on leadership skills are filed in the leadership and management section. Other reflective notes concerning less readily categorised experiences can then be filed in a dedicated section (e.g. dealing with conduct problems in colleagues or attending court). If this method is chosen, then a contents page will still be useful and it would be a matter of judgement as to whether to list all reflective notes in the portfolio and where to find them, or refer to only those filed in that section.

Difficult-to-evidence competencies and reflective practice

The key components of reflective practice from the point of view of appraisal are:

- that a professional issue or situation is clearly described
- what action the individual took or did not take
- what went well
- what could be done differently to produce a better outcome
- what needs to be learned in order to achieve this better outcome.

The reflective notes completed as examples in this book reflect these basic requirements. There are certain domains within the competency-based curriculum that appear hard to evidence; commonly these include health and probity. However, on further consideration very common problems that practising doctors encounter routinely fall under these domains and can be reflected on in just the same way, with the resulting reflections recorded on a form contributing as portfolio evidence. Examples of this might include the ethics of seeing drug representatives or receiving gifts from patients for probity and being deprived of sleep or being stressed at work for health.

Example of a poor reflection

Box 6.2 provides an example of a poor reflection. It is poor as it simply describes an event that has taken place. It does not think about areas for learning or improvement. A better reflection may have thought about the difficulties in accessing physical care for psychiatric in-patients and what might be done to bridge the gap.

Example of a good reflection

Box 6.3 provides an example of a good reflection. This reflection demonstrates clearly what was learned, how the outcome could be improved next time and what further learning and experiences are required. The account also discusses feedback that was received. Feedback may be written under a separate subheading in the reflective piece. Some reflective accounts will also give consideration to how the experience affected the trainee or the team. This should be included if it aids learning.

Box 6.2 Example of a poor reflection

Give a brief description of this experience

Part of my duties is to monitor physical health needs of the patients. This requires the ability to undertake physical examination of patients and investigate them appropriately (e.g. blood tests).

On some occasions, examination and/or carrying out and interpreting investigative tests have led me to make the decision to transfer patients to the medical wards at the infirmary for appropriate treatment (e.g. intravenous antibiotics for pneumonia). Similarly, some patients have become delirious with, for example, urinary tract infections, and this has required appropriate investigation (e.g. midstream urine samples) and treatment.

What did you learn?

That I am able to safely look after patients' physical health needs. I am able to recognise when I require help from other specialists, such as knowing when it is appropriate to transfer a patient to a medical or surgical ward or when to discuss the patient with medics/surgeons.

Box 6.3 Example of a good reflection

Give a brief description of this experience

The crisis resolution and home treatment (CRHT) team asked for an urgent medication review of a patient who had been recently discharged from the ward. He had moderate depression and generalised anxiety. The crisis team nurse said she felt that the patient was worse than before admission; particularly noticeable was his low mood and loss of weight.

A CRHT team member told me that she wanted to change the patient's antidepressant to mirtazepine and also to start quetiapine for his anxiety. She told me she had done the nurse prescribing course and that if she had her PIN number, she would have made the changes anyway.

I thought that the medication review could wait another day until the staff grade was back, but the CRHT team were adamant that I see the patient that day. I went to the patient's home with a different team member. The patient expressed his concerns that citalopram and diazepam were not adequate and that he felt something needed to be done.

I was under pressure from the patient and the CRHT team member to make a decision. I therefore negotiated that we would start quetiapine and wean off diazepam in the hope of improving anxiety symptoms and ultimately helping the depression.

I was then able to run this past the staff grade 2 days later. He disagreed with this management, saying that the antidepressant should have been changed instead. He told me that changing the antidepressant is more evidence based in managing the depression and anxiety rather than using an antipsychotic.

What did you learn?

I learned that I should stand my ground about making a decision I'm not comfortable with.

I've learned about changing antidepressants when discussing the case with the staff grade.

I've learned that sometimes 'urgent' medication reviews can wait 24 h (unless of course the patient is expressing frank suicidal ideation or is at any other great risk – that was not the case here).

How will you amend your PDP in the light of this experience?

I need to learn about managing anxiety, especially with comorbid depression. I will read up on this using the *Oxford Textbook of Psychiatry* and look to gain more experience with these patients in the community.

I need to read a review article on the use of antipsychotics in treating anxiety, so that I understand the evidence base and rationale for their use.

Key points to remember

- The successful portfolio must contain a good amount of reflective practice relating to both clinical and non-clinical experience.
- Reflective notes should cover the nature of the experience, any feedback, lessons learned, and how these inform professional development.
- Trainees must decide how to make reflective notes more informative either by filing them in a separate section of the portfolio or filing them where relevant, or a combination of these approaches.

CHAPTER 7

Audit and research

This chapter relates to experience and competence concerning audit, research, publications, posters and presentations, and how to best present this work. Everybody's PDP should contain an element of research, and trainees are usually expected to complete at least one audit annually. A key point to remember here is to be orderly and present audit in the audit section and research in the research section: there is nothing more frustrating for the academically minded psychiatrist than when audit and research are confused with each other.

Audit

Clinical audit is a quality improvement process which aims to better outcomes. Usually this would be done through aiming to meet pre-determined standards.

As one's career develops, one, hopefully, becomes increasingly experienced and autonomous with audit ideas and projects. It may be valuable to start with a short statement of acquired skills with respect to audit, personal views on the role of audit in mental health services and the psychiatric trainee's role with reference to what the curriculum requires and how this contributes to professional development planning. The portfolio demonstrates trainees' current level of ability and experience. With this in mind, it might be useful to present work in context of experience and past projects. Therefore, one method of presenting audit experience might be in chronological order:

- personal audit history (shows track record)
- current audit(s) (as required)
- planned audits or ideas (shows acquisition of skills, PDP, etc.).

Give a brief abstract for each audit such that the reader knows exactly what has been done and what skills were involved, including personal level of involvement, method, results and any changes or improvements that have occurred as a result. A hypothetical example of how this might look is provided in Box 7.1.

Box 7.1 Example of an audit abstract

Audits of the completion of Section 136 forms

Royal Anthorn Hospital, 2010

Background: A number of recent complaints where made about the absence of the required documents after assessments following the police implementing their holding power.

Involvement: I planned and co-conducted this audit project with the psychiatric liaison nurses. I created the data collection sheet with assistance of the audit department.

Method: Data were collected retrospectively for a 2-year period. Records were scrutinised from medical records and the Mental Health Act administrator.

Main findings: Paper work was only found for 20% of cases in the above period, of a total of 56, and was generally incomplete. It was found that at least five detentions occurred without any written record of the fact.

Improvements: Educational meetings conducted by liaison staff were provided for accident and emergency staff and at the local police station. Practice is to be re-audited in 6 months' time.

In this example it is very clear what the reasons for the audit were, the involvement of the trainee and any outcomes as a result. All audits may not be impressive or groundbreaking but the format shown in Box 7.1 allows trainees to effectively communicate the necessary information easily and succinctly. The ARCP and appointment panels are particularly interested when trainees are able to close the audit cycle, particularly when they are able to show improvement. It must be remembered that reporting even a successful audit does not necessarily evidence one's competence in completing a project. Reflective notes about the reasons for the audit, better approaches to execution and the value of findings and improving practice better evidence a trainee's competence in audit.

At the end of the audit section it may also be helpful to provide full copies of audit reports, depending on the particulars of the project itself.

Research

Not all trainees will be published researchers, indeed it is probably the minority that do. However, the PDP should always contain an element of research. The required type of experience and level of attainment in research will depend on your level of seniority and this will naturally increase over time. It is vital that in terms of planning for a year in training, trainees must refer themselves to the curriculum and competency list to make sure they understand what is required and give themselves enough time to plan out projects and courses. Here, we will consider how to manage the material as well as providing suggestions as to how to gain experience.

For those trainees with actual project experience and publication

Trainees differ widely in the amount of research experience they will gain. For those trainees who have actual project experience, with or without some form of publication, it is important to consider the presentation of this experience in the context of the portfolio. It should be remembered that research takes an enormous amount of planning, revising, literature searching, data collection, analysis, writing up and endless re-drafting, and it would be easy to fall into the trap of presenting too much information. In terms of research, what does the reader need to know in order to understand trainees' level of competence with respect to research? The reader should be able to gain an impression of the answer to this question quite quickly. Trainees should understand their developmental needs using the following prompts and use them to inform the structure of the presentation of work.

- What does the curriculum require you to evidence?
- What are your skills or exactly what have you done (e.g. planning, creating data collection sheets, training in semi-structured interviews, skills with statistical analysis and computer programs, writing papers, achieving publication)?
- What projects have you been involved with and what was your level of involvement (e.g. naturalistic studies, cross-sectional epidemiology, randomised controlled trials, reviews)?
- How were the results of your research disseminated or published (e.g. local posters, national posters, international conferences, journal articles that are peer reviewed, letters to the editor)?

These prompting questions should be tracked on to the curricular requirements. The ARCP is about demonstrating that trainees have met the competencies described in the curriculum for that stage of training, such that requirements will be different in the first year compared with the last. With these questions in mind, trainees able to report experience and projects might consider a three-tiered approach to presenting their work. This system should allow readers an increasing insight into trainees' skills and experience, being able to refer themselves to full articles if necessary but at the same time not becoming overwhelmed. This allows trainees to see in what areas they need to develop next.

A summary of experience

This summary should very briefly detail work completed, including the fact of publication or presentation. This should look something like the example in Box 7.2.

> **Box 7.2 Example of a summary of experience**
>
> **Dr JS Baker**
>
> *Summary of research experience*
>
> Baker JS, Collins R, Peters C (2010) Do GPs agree with psychiatrist diagnoses following GP initiated referral? A 1-day survey of inner city GPs. *Psychiatry*, **36**, 112–6.
>
> Baker JS, *et al* (2009) *Demographic factors and the use of the nurses holding power*. Unpublished.
>
> Tooley J, Dearlove B, Jacobs D, Baker JS (2008) *Can we be confident in offering mood stabilisers to patients with borderline personality disorder. A review*. Poster Presentation at the Royal College of Psychiatrists International Congress, London, 2006.

Statements and abstracts

Before providing abstracts it can be useful to include a basic statement or summary regarding research skills. This should be brief, four to six sentences, and should cover the following aspects:

- skills and areas for development
- the types of research projects in which you have experience
- the role of the psychiatrist as a researcher
- how you reflect on your academic skills, integrate them in clinical practice and expand on them.

A brief statement like this will give a good overview of your stage of development, current level of skills and experience, evidence of development planning, an impression of reflective practice and as a driver to further development.

In this next section trainees can proceed to provide a structured abstract for each project that answers all four prompting questions suggested on p. 41. These abstracts should be presented in the same order as suggested in the summary list. The format for the abstracts is at your discretion as long as you address the prompts. The example in Box 7.3 does this.

Attaching feedback to these summaries will help to demonstrate competence. This might include some form of WPBA or other written feedback, a self-reflective piece or a self-recorded evaluation of learning that includes feedback from more experienced colleagues.

Full articles

In this last section, trainees have the option to file copies of the original journal articles, unpublished manuscripts, posters and presentations. These should also be placed in the order in which they appear in the summary list. They are then available for the reader should they wish to examine them in more detail, or refer to a specific part.

Box 7.3 Example of a structured abstract for a project

Title: Do GPs agree with psychiatric diagnoses following GP-initiated referral? A 1-day survey of inner-city GPs.

Authors: Baker JS, Collins R & Peters C.

Background: It is known that diagnoses made by general practitioners (GPs) are often divergent from those made by psychiatrists. It is not known what views GPs take on diagnoses made by psychiatrists on patients they have themselves referred for an opinion.

Method: A 1-day survey was sent out to all GPs in inner-city Manchester; this was conducted on paper and electronically according to the GP's preference. General practitioners were asked to record their opinions regarding the diagnoses made, concerning the last ten referrals they made to psychiatrists. Diagnoses, demographics and risk issues where recorded.

Results: GPs disputed diagnoses made by psychiatrists in almost 40% of cases; in the majority of cases, psychiatrists diagnosed personality disorder when GPs diagnosed depression or psychosis. This disparity was associated with risk to others and suicide as well as being more frequent when the patients where under the age of 35.

Conclusions: GPs and psychiatrists will often not reach the same diagnosis; GPs dispute this particularly regarding those younger patients they perceive to have psychosis or depression. Further research is needed to establish how GPs and psychiatrists are making diagnoses. This would establish the need to revise this aspect of training.

Personal involvement and skills: I joined this project in the late planning stage but contributed to revisions of plans. I created the data collection forms and collected data with other researchers. I analysed the data with help form a medical statistician and drafted the method and results section. I co-drafted the conclusions. During this time we had to overcome resistance to participate and consider the logistics of resources available.

Dissemination/publication: *Psychiatry*, 2010, **36**, 112–6. This is a peer-reviewed article.

For those trainees with limited or no project experience

The method of presenting experience detailed in the previous section applies if trainees have completed projects to present. The reality is that a large number of trainees will not have work of this type to present. Research and academic skills can still be evidenced if trainees are creative and give some thought to what must be demonstrated in terms of competence, underlying the need for careful reference to the curriculum. Below are some suggestions that could apply. This is not an exhaustive list. It is stressed that these should clearly relate to competencies and should be well indexed in the summary of evidence, so that the reader can clearly understand its relevance and what it contributes as evidence to. Trainees with research experience may also wish to further evidence their skills and experience.

- Attend research meetings – consider contacting academic psychiatrists and other researchers and ask to attend meetings. This will allow trainees to observe and contribute to the running and execution of established research projects. Researchers are often pleased of assistance, especially with data collection or analysis – if trainees are asked to help, they need to be clear on the educational value of the task. It would be especially valuable for those who trainees observe or work with to provide feedback, commenting on competencies, contributions and skills. Such experience should prompt the recording of reflective practice.

- Courses – these need to be appropriate to the level of skills for the current stage of training. Shorter courses on basic literature searching and advanced searching are valuable: check to see whether the course is certified. Such courses are sometimes available online. Courses and seminars are also available concerning research methodology; again, record a good account of the educational content and get a certificate of attendance. It is stressed that attending a course and having a certificate on its own is not evidence of competence; however, it could be used as a basis of self-appraisal and reflective practice.

- Local journal clubs – these can be quite valuable. Journal clubs will cover a range of research methodologies, with critique. Adding a brief educational talk about a particular research method prior to an article presentation would be a good demonstration of your understanding. You could link these to WPBAs including Assessment of Teaching and Journal Club Presentations.

- Draft a research protocol – even if you do not have the time or resources available, you could still draft a project protocol that covers the important aspects of methodology, ethical approval and statistical analysis. This could be discussed with your educational supervisor or another appropriate professional; this is all the more helpful if you receive written feedback. Although this does not mean you actually conduct a project, it does demonstrate that you are aware of the scientific principles and procedures.

Key points to remember

- As a starting point, check early on exactly what competencies you need to evidence – planning is key.
- For those with projects, present these in brief and then in detail, making it clear what your skills are and what was your involvement in the project.
- If trainees have not been involved in research, academic skills can be evidenced in a variety of ways, including simple approaches such as journal clubs.

CHAPTER 8

Teaching

Teaching forms a large part of the competencies trainees need to demonstrate – especially as trainees become more senior – and is yet another role that the psychiatrist can reasonably be expected to fulfil.

Teaching can occur in a variety of situations, indirectly (e.g. shadowing by a medical student) or directly (e.g. giving a formal teaching session on the mental state examination to foundation doctors). There are therefore many opportunities in which a trainee can act as a teacher, record experience, be assessed and thus demonstrate competency. There are also courses which a trainee can attend, such as to become a communication skills tutor or to become an examiner. Examining and assessing is another important skill to develop. When planning teaching, trainees should always refer to the curriculum to ensure that this will enable development and evidence of the relevant competencies. It is valuable to plan how evidence of competency will be recorded, for example by recording topics or the use of WPBAs such as Journal Club Presentation, Case Presentation or Assessment of Teaching.

As with other areas of the portfolio, this section should record exactly what teaching has been undertaken and what skills are involved. This should follow the format:

- a clear explanation of the task and topic
- the skills required and the application of any previous training
- a reference to content
- assessments, feedback and reflection.

Reflecting on what went well and what could be done better is always valuable, especially if it adds to your professional development. Trainees may therefore wish to link the assessment or experience to a reflective note. Box 8.1 is an example of how a trainee might present their work.

Box 8.1 Example of linking an assessment to a reflective note

Group composition/size: Third-year medical students
Venue: Medical education centre   Session duration: 45 min

	Significantly short of competence at ST3 level	Approaching competence at ST3 level	Competent at ST3 level
1 Material preparation	✓		
2 Environment preparation		✓	
3 Structure			✓
4 Presentation and delivery			✓
5 Quality of aids		✓	
6 Appropriateness of aids		✓	
7 Use of aids		✓	
8 Answering questions			✓
9 Overall rating		✓	

Anything particularly good?
Conversational and interactive style. Putting open questions back to the audience.

Any areas for development?
Some of the slides were very wordy and as such hard to read quickly at the same time as paying attention to you as the presenter.

Agreed action
To give this session again at the next intake of students but revise the slides as suggested.

Reflective note: self-appraisal of learning
Brief description of learning of this experience
I was assessed by my supervisor giving a 45 min presentation to a group of six third-year medical students on an introduction to psychiatry as a part of their third-year mind and movement modules. I had prepared this against their curriculum and learning needs for the attachment.

What did you learn?
I found the session flowed much better when I allowed short silences to happen and putting questions to the group to try and help them feel involved in the session.

What feedback did you get from your assessor?
Positive in the main in terms of content and delivery but some of my slides where a bit too long and might have been distracting from my talking.

I also looked at the feedback forms completed by the audience. They echoed the feedback from my supervisor – generally positive but slides too wordy.

In light of this experience, what do you need to learn about, and how will you adapt your PDP?
I am going to give this talk again, but between now and then I will take my slides to one of my colleagues with an interest in education and ask them for any further suggestions about using slides and specific observations about this talk. I will then revise the talk.

Key points to remember

- Presentation of teaching experience should communicate the task, topics, teaching methods, skills, feedback and assessment.
- Teaching experience should be planned according to curriculum competencies appropriate to the individual's stage in training.

CHAPTER 9

Psychotherapy experience

Psychotherapeutic skills and experience within different schools of therapy remain an important part of training. The portfolio should therefore not simply record the fact of courses, training and experience in a certain area, but should also detail knowledge, skills and attitudes in this respect and how they have been integrated into competent practice.

Recording activity and competence

Over the course of 3 years' basic training, trainees should build up a catalogue of experience. Presenting an account of this is part of demonstrating development and will usually include:

- previous Balint group involvement
- interview skills training
- specific forms of therapy, including cognitive–behavioural therapy, cognitive analytic therapy and psychodynamic therapy with associated feedback
- training days or courses
- other specific experience.

During the years of core training, trainees need to demonstrate a level of general psychological competence. This essentially entails being able to account for clinical phenomena in psychological terms, demonstrating advanced communication skills and advanced emotional intelligence in dealings with patients and colleagues. At later stages, this will more specifically involve demonstrating appropriate referral for formal psychotherapies, jointly managing patients receiving psychotherapy and delivering basic psychotherapeutic treatments and strategies where appropriate.

At the time of writing the minimum requirements for demonstrating acquisition of the competencies at CT3 level are:

1 Attend a minimum of 30 CbD groups over the first 12–18 months of core training and provide evidence of the attainment of appropriate competencies through the use of the CbD tool.

2   Undertake two psychotherapy cases in two modalities and over two different durations between years CT1 and CT3. (Trainees must achieve the competencies in the CbD groups, usually by the end of CT1, before proceeding to undertaking psychotherapy cases under supervision.)

3   Complete a psychotherapy ACE for each of the different modalities of psychotherapy undertaken.

More detailed and up-to-date information on psychotherapy competencies and training requirements can be found on the Royal College of Psychiatrists' website: www.rcpsych.ac.uk/specialties/faculties/ psychotherapy/training.aspx.

It is helpful to provide details of what psychotherapy experience has involved. This could potentially become very long-winded but the record itself should be orderly and informative. It might be helpful to follow the 'Who? Where? Why? When? and What?' format of questioning to complete this. It may also be helpful to have this section follow in chronological order; this provides a framework, a place to start and shows how trainees are developing. Because this type of information can easily become unwieldy and hard to digest, one suggestion could be a shortlist of experience followed by a longer description of each example in more detail on separate pages.

An example of presenting psychotherapy experience

First, provide a shortlist in chronological order (Box 9.1). Although this list is not in itself very informative, it does give a preliminary overview about which areas trainees have experience in, what is planned and which areas are yet to be covered – a developmental overview.

The next stage would be to expand on the shortlist to provide a more detailed summary of each experience. It is helpful to summarise each area into a standardised format. This has a number of advantages: it improves presentation of work, ensures the recording of all relevant information

---

Box 9.1 Example of presentation of psychotherapy experience

Summary of experience in psychotherapy to date

- Interview skills training, August 2007 to September 2008
- Balint group (closed), August 2007 to Jaury 2009
- Psychodynamic skills group, August 2008 to January 2009
- Psychodynamic psychotherapy short case, February 2009 to August 2009
- Psychodynamic psychotherapy long case, August 2009 to present
- Cognitive–behavioural therapy introduction course, February 2010
- Cognitive–behavioural therapy case, expected start date August 2010

and remains reader-friendly despite the fact that towards the end of core training trainees will have a great deal of experience and skills in this area.

Table 9.1 is a hypothetical example and the information given is fictional. The format is not important as long as it conveys the information necessary to understand what has actually occurred and the skills involved.

It is clear that although this summary does not cover the entirety of what was done and achieved in therapy and does not in itself demonstrate competence, it does give an account of the aims, skills and techniques used.

CbD groups in psychotherapeutic aspects of psychiatry

Year 1 and/or year 2 core trainees should attend one of these groups on a weekly basis, where psychotherapeutic issues relating to clinical work are discussed. A record of satisfactory attendance and participation should be kept in the portfolio along with CbD group assessment WPBA forms completed after 6 months and 12 months attendance at the group. These forms should be presented as evidence of satisfactory attainment of competencies at the first or second ARCP.

Structured Assessment of Psychotherapy Expertise (SAPE)

This WPBA is completed by the supervisor based on their experience of trainees' performance. These are completed after finishing therapy in a recognised modality, when a brief 500-word summary is presented. Standards refer to level of performance expected by CT3.

Other WPBA forms

There have been other assessment forms devised to assess psychotherapeutic skills. If you choose to use these, it should be stressed that it would be wise to consider them as further evidence in addition to what is suggested above and not to rely on them alone if they are not formally approved by your deanery or, if you are in England, your local education and training board (LETB).

Reflective practice

Reflective notes add another level of depth to the psychotherapy section of the portfolio, as they demonstrate how trainees are able to identify useful skills and techniques that improve their practice. Reflective notes also demonstrates aspects of emotional intelligence, points of reflection that may occur during therapy or in supervision as well as in discussion groups, and are all valuable. It is the decision of the individual as to where

Table 9.1 A detailed example of psychotherapy experience

Therapy type	Cognitive–behavioural therapy
Patient details, problems and goals of therapy	A 28-year-old professional man with social phobia. We aimed to enable him to chair meetings at work and reduce his use of short-term anxiolytic medication.
Dates of therapy, frequency of sessions and number of sessions	Therapy commenced 28 March 2010 and ended 12 June 2010. We met weekly and completed 11 sessions, with 1 follow-up session 8 weeks following end of therapy.
Supervision type Name of supervisor(s)	Supervision occurred on a 1:1 basis with Dr Bronson, consultant psychiatrist and cognitive–behavioural therapist.
Summary of therapy and techniques involved	Session 1 and 2 were used to produce a formulation. I used diagrams with the patient's words to produce a cross-sectional cycle, which help him to add further descriptors to our formulation. We built on a rough formulation he did as homework after our first session. Sessions 3–9: These include a number of in-session and out-of-session behavioural experiments. We used predictions to interpret the results of the experiments and graphical scales to challenge cognitive distortions. When the outcome of experiments was unproductive, we went back to check our formulation and then refined it according to the automatic thought and ways in which we could improve the usefulness of the exercise. Sessions 10 and 11 were used to summarise our progress as part of the relapse prevention work. Session 12: This was a follow-up session. The patient was functioning well. He brought back one instance of a social situation that he felt did not go well. We looked at our formulation and identified some alternative coping strategies.
Summary of issues discussed in supervision	Initially, we reviewed our formulation and highlighted areas where more detail was needed. Later, we looked at how the formulation can be used to inform behavioural experiments. We discussed the use of scaling to challenge cognitive distortions as this seemed to fit the patient's thinking style. We reviewed the results of a behavioural experiment that did not go as planned and seemed to support the patient's negative view of themselves. We looked at this, relating it to the initial formulation and thinking of different ways of looking at the results. We discussed the value of re-running a well-planned experiment in the presence of a strong formulation and good therapeutic alliance and the inevitability of setbacks.
Learning from experience, reflections and changes to practice	A robust formulation guides the content of therapy, spending the time to get this right is valuable. Homework experiments outside therapy may not always go according to plan and have negative consequences, managing setbacks in therapy can be one of the key skills. Some therapeutic skills such as recognising and challenging automatic thoughts are useful in my day-to-day clinical practice.

they want to file any psychotherapy WPBAs or reflective notes, be this in the psychotherapy section, WPBA section or a separate reflective practice section. It would be wise to give the location of any relevant assessment or reflective notes in the psychotherapy section if they are filed elsewhere.

Psychotherapy competencies for year 4–6 specialist trainees (ST4–6)

The requirements are different for each specialty. Undertaking psychotherapy cases may not be necessary (although this can be done if it is trainees' interest), for example in general adult training. Therefore competencies must be demonstrated in other ways. Competencies would include knowing when to refer for psychological therapy and which therapies would be of benefit or contraindicated in certain patients. An ability to explain therapies is important. Trainees will also need to be able to evaluate the outcome of psychological therapies and provide aftercare and appropriate management alongside therapy. Here are some possible ways to demonstrate this:

- CbD (with a psychologist or psychotherapist) of a patient with challenging difficulties which may require a psychological formulation
- attendance at meetings regarding local psychological services (e.g. commissioning of new services or re-structuring)
- attendance at community mental health team allocation meetings when a psychologist is present
- many courses and teaching sessions are available
- journal clubs which review evidence of psychotherapeutic techniques
- reflective practice (e.g. when you have referred a patient for psychotherapy and reflect on the outcome).

Whichever method is used, there should be a description of how the experience or learning has further developed the trainee's competency, according to the curriculum. There should also be a reflection of what further learning needs have been identified to attain competency or to develop it further.

Key points to remember

- Start with a brief chronological list of experience.
- Give details of each area of psychotherapy experience in a standardised format that clearly communicates timescales, skills and techniques.
- Use some method of linking your experience to reflective practice including aspects of emotional self-awareness and intelligence.

CHAPTER 10

Management and leadership experience

Management and leadership are two of the many duties of a doctor, and this is no less the case for the psychiatrist. Although more senior management experience is more relevant to trainees towards the end of their training, every trainee's portfolio should contain an element of management experience.

The portfolio is competency driven and although a list of experience shows that trainees are engaging in some level of management experience, it does not demonstrate performance. Leadership occurs in many situations, so time should be taken to think creatively, within reason, about what experience is sought and how it is presented.

What to communicate about management experience and skills

The training portfolio will benefit from a description of what actually occurred and what the developmental issues are. It may be helpful to consider the following questions in brief:

- What does the curriculum require in terms of management competencies?
- What was your role and who formed part of the team?
- What were the challenges or issues?
- What were the barriers to good team working?
- How were setbacks overcome?
- What skills were needed to be successful?
- What were the developmental needs following this experience?
- What type of feedback was given and what did it say?

Consider the following list of experience that a trainee might present.

1 Doctors in training representative for trainees CT1–3.
2 Rota coordinator.
3 Observer at consultant meetings.

As experience all these are perfectly good examples but on their own they do not detail experience and development. Contrast this list with Box 10.1 and how the brief paragraph covers the prompts suggested.

Presenting experience in this way and linking that to reflective notes and key learning points makes this part of the portfolio much more informative and developmental. Other methods of demonstrating leadership experience might include the following.

- A personal statement concerning the doctor's role as a manager, describing individual skills and how these have been integrated by reflective practice.
- It may be worthwhile adding a reflective note about each experience further capitalising on this part of skills and experience in a manner appropriate to the portfolio. This could be done in a similar way as suggested with WPBAs (see Chapter 5).

Box 10.1 Example of list of experience and corresponding explanations

1 Doctors in training representative for trainees CT1–3

I was elected as representative. We met every 2 weeks and I would chair meetings. Here we would consider any problems with access to trainers, educational supervision, completing WPBAs and uncertainties regarding the ARCP. I needed to give everyone a chance to speak but keep order in the meetings. I would need to convey any problems to the college tutor or the deanery and at times act as a go-between, trying to balance trainees' expectations and what the scheme can reasonably provide. This required time for me to reflect on the issues and seek supervision as necessary. I learned the importance of timely and sensitive communication of trainees' concerns to the appropriate person.

2 Rota coordinator

After putting myself forward as rota coordinator I arranged a first meeting with all doctors on the rota to get everyone around the table and ensure the rota is covered for 6 months. There was a delicate balance between ensuring the service was covered and considering an individual's personal needs. This required sensitivity to cultural issues and facilitating amicable compromise between colleagues. During this time I facilitated a consultation period with medical staff regarding changes to the rota following the European Working Time Directive, gaining an insight into the implementation of health and safety legislation.

3 Observer at consultant meetings

During the 6 months in in-patient services I sat in on monthly consultant meetings. These covered areas such as consultation with new policies and the trust's position on prescribing. Often members of higher management such as the executive directors attended and the results of clinical audit were discussed. I gained insight to how findings from local audit translate into changes in practice, which often included resolution of differing views between consultants on the best way to proceed. I learned about the balance between clinical need, policy and resource availability.

- Could another lead/member of the team provide feedback about team-working skills with reference to observed performance? It may be worth referring them to the curriculum before they put pen to paper, increasing the relevance of any document to evidence of competence.
- Some deaneries may offer leadership courses aimed at higher trainees, for example a 'medical leadership in practice' course which teaches theory and supports trainees in undertaking a leadership project. These courses may be in collaboration with a university and can potentially lead to higher training such as a Masters in medical leadership or health policy.

Key points to remember

- Bear in mind that experience and skills also need to relate to competencies in the curriculum.
- Provide a brief description of the experience, what skills were needed and what was learned.
- Link experience with reflective practice.

CHAPTER 11

Appraisal reports, planning meetings and educational objectives

Plans and reports

Some plans and appraisals are required as part of the portfolio and the completion of the ARCP. In a dedicated section, these reports should start with a contents page and include:

- initial planning meeting
- PDP
- mid-point review
- educational supervisor's reports
- college tutor's structured report or training programme director's report
- completing the annual GMC survey is usually mandatory and evidence of its completion should be included in the portfolio
- some specialties in some deaneries may also require an annual survey to be completed for more specific feedback.

If individual deaneries do not have specific forms for these, they are available from the Royal College of Psychiatrists. Remember to make best use of these reports – they contain reference to competencies and should be signed; they therefore can contribute to evidence of competence.

Records of on-call work and educational supervision

Recording of previous placements, current placement and duties is required. Trainees should also record the nature of their current clinical activities and on-call/emergency work. Details of supervision with educational supervisors should also be recorded. This can be a very useful forum for discussion on issues pertaining to competencies that are harder to evidence; for example, a discussion about what happens in the event of a patient dying or working with the coroner. This is especially helpful if the supervisor has signed a formal record of supervision.

The format used to record these meetings and activities is not as important as conveying the required information. It is stressed that trainees must demonstrate an achievable and relevant set of educational objectives and that these relate to competencies relevant to the stage of training. It is therefore important that trainees take the curriculum to planning meetings with educational supervisors so that development planning is targeted and relevant. Table 11.1 illustrates how the information presented can be valuable in terms of use as evidence of competence.

Table 11.1 Record of on-call activity

Case description	Learning points	Validation (supervisors signature)
03/06/2010 Advice given to orthopaedics specialist registrar who wanted to refer a patient with schizophrenia who would not return home claiming sexual abuse was occurring at the hands of her fellow tenants. I advised on the basis of the information available that if there are not acute 'psychiatric concerns' (no suicidal or violent acts or thoughts, no affective or psychotic disorder) that their concerns must be addressed and taken seriously, as if not she may well be at risk and ignoring her would be discrimination. Advised on proceeding on engaging Social Services. Also advised that Mental Capacity Act 2005 is only of limited help and they are not looking at a treatment decision.	Discussed with consultant, correct advice regarding legal position and protocols as well as advocating for the patient. Suggestions for development: to look at safeguarding vulnerable adults procedures for the locality and consider e-learning on the College website on the same.	JS Lorenson

---

Key points to remember

- There a number of reports that are required.
- Plan your educational objectives early with reference to competencies.
- Use other records, such as records of supervision, to further evidence competencies.

CHAPTER 12

Other experiences, achievements and documents

An additional, perhaps miscellaneous section, can be useful for experiences, documents or achievements that simply do not fit elsewhere in the portfolio but are of use in contributing towards evidence. The guiding principle here should be why is this in the portfolio and what competency does this relate to? This is an important point and needs emphasis. A degree certificate is certainly an achievement but alone it is not evidence of competence. The list of what could conceivably be included in this section is endless and the following examples are intended as a guide to illustrate how various documents can be used.

Certificates

- Original degree
- Other degree certificates
- GMC certificate
- Disclosure and Barring Service clearance
- Intermediate and basic life support
- Breakaway techniques certificate
- MRCPsych exams (some people give number of attempts)

Although these may not relate directly to specific competencies, they do say something about level of seniority and staying up to date. If any of these are related to competency, a word about their content should be given. For example, if it is a certificate concerning an examined course, a brief note about the content of the course, the skills involved, key learning points, reflective notes and the fact of the examination should be added. This should then be indexed in the summary of evidence section, especially if it involves any directly observed skills in practice. As most training schemes and NHS trusts require annual breakaway and cardiopulmonary resuscitation training, why not also use these to complete a DOPS (Direct Observation of Procedural Skills) WPBA?

Your curriculum vitae

The curriculum vitae (CV) may appear slightly outdated now with the electronic application system for jobs and the existence of the portfolio itself. The CV can be useful if it can be structured with competencies in mind. It can further be used as a bank for achievements you may have that do not fit well into the portfolio. It should be remembered that the portfolio contains evidence of competence, so unsubstantiated claims are not helpful. Therefore, and for example, a section of the CV concerning awards with a list of prizes for clinical excellence only becomes evidence when accompanied with the supporting documentation. Some members of the ARCP panel may well take the view that a CV alone is not evidence of anything and may not take it into account. A further point to consider is that it is important to avoid padding out the portfolio unnecessarily – selective evidence is key.

Letters of thanks or acknowledgement

These may come from patients or colleagues; they can serve as less formal evidence of the relationships formed in the workplace. They will have an explicit content as well as an implicit message about trainees. If these are included, it should be ensured that it is made clear what competency they relate to and confidentiality must always be observed.

What about health and probity?

These domains are critical to practice and public confidence in the profession and yet trainees often struggle to demonstrate their good practice in these respects. In the first instance this should be seen as a good thing if, in the year in training, there have been no concerns about the trainee's probity or health. However, this, superficially at least, leaves trainees with a problem: what do I reflect on? The following are common and reasonable examples.

Health

- Have you attended the GP in the last year?
- Have you bypassed the normal NHS referral systems?
- Do you have a long-term condition?
- Do you have coping strategies for stress?
- Do you actively self-care?

Your reflections should focus on a description of the issue, whether and how this has affected you at work, and what you might need to do differently to manage things better in the future.

Probity

- The ethics of seeing pharmaceutical representatives
- Telling patients which pharmacist to use
- Accepting gifts from patients
- Colleagues underperforming or ill at work
- When to breach confidentiality

Your reflections should include a brief description of the matter, what was good about your actions, what was less good about your actions and what you will do next time based on your learning as well as any learning needs identified.

If the suggestions above still do not help to generate reflections, real GMC fitness to practice cases relating to health and probity are published publicly and are readily available. Trainees can always read these cases, discuss them at peer groups or with supervisors and record their reflections. For further reading and insights relating to health and probity, you might want to read *Evidence for Medical Appraisal* (National Association of Primary Care Educators & Clinical Governance Support Team, 2007).

Key point to remember

- There are a number of additional documents or achievements that can be valuable in the portfolio but remember that the curriculum is competency based, therefore explain anything you present – what exactly did you do, what are your skills?

Further reading

National Association of Primary Care Educators & Clinical Governance Support Team (2007) *Evidence for Medical Appraisal: Essential/Optional. Statement of the NAPCE/CGST Conference.* NAPCE/CGST. Available from http://www.revalidationsupport.nhs.uk/responsible_officer/responsible_officer_links/ROlinksdocumentarchive.php.

CHAPTER 13

The future of portfolios

In all likelihood, portfolios are here to stay. They provide a system to demonstrate competency and therefore public accountability. With the introduction of revalidation by the GMC, all doctors at all levels need to be appraised and portfolios are required for this (General Medical Council, 2013). Trainees' appraisal for revalidation will take place at the ARCP panel. It is most likely that all organisations (deaneries (LETBs as of April 2013 in England), NHS trusts and private healthcare providers) will move to e-portfolios, as there are pedagogical gains as well as being easier to administrate (Strivens *et al*, 2009). The case is put forward that a well-maintained portfolio will ensure public accountability (Ingrassia, 2013).

Keeping a portfolio may help doctors identify areas of interest and keep a 'portfolio career'. This may increase job satisfaction and reduce burnout if doctors take on interests such as management, medical education, research, medico-legal work or even media, business, humanitarian aid or health policy. This will also reduce absence through sickness and increase productivity (Pathiraja & Wilson, 2011).

Medical Royal Colleges, deaneries or schools (i.e. specialties) within deaneries may have designed a portfolio which is being used. Some trainees may get frustrated with it, or identify ways to improve it without necessarily being able to influence change. There is no consistency, either between portfolios or deaneries/LETBs, so expectations can be different. The future may be a standardised portfolio (which would make writing guides such as this easier) or even a fluid, ever-evolving portfolio which is an open source so that trainees and educationalists in deaneries can modify it. This has the benefit of the potential for majority rule. An open-source portfolio has been proposed and is in its embryonic stages at the time of writing (see http://oportfol.io).

The *BMJ* have made a portfolio app, which allows the user to document clinical encounters and e-learning. However, it does not yet integrate with the portfolio which this book describes in detail. Integration of e-portofolios with apps is beginning to take place in non-medical areas, for example: https://sites.google.com/site/eportfolioapps/.

Twitter is being used as a platform for collaborating and troubleshooting the foundation doctor e-portofolio. This allows the flow of ideas and the potential to gain national consensus to drive up consistency and standards (e.g. https://twitter.com/NESePortfolio). There is an app available for use with this portfolio (https://app.nhseportfolios.org/app), but access requires a password so we could not assess its functionality.

Whatever the future, portfolios will be there, and likely with increasing use of technology. Doctors will have to ensure that they are able to plan time into their working week to use their portfolio, and to learn while doing so. We owe it to our patients.

References

General Medical Council (2013) *Ready for Revalidation: The Good Medical Practice Framework for Appraisal and Revalidation*. GMC.

Ingrassia A (2013) Portfolio-based learning in medical education. *Advances in Psychiatric Treatment*, **19**, 329–36.

Pathiraja F, Wilson MC (2011) The rise and rise of the portfolio career. *BMJ Careers*, 19 January (http://careers.bmj.com/careers/advice/view-article.html?id=20001807).

Strivens J, Baume D, Grant S, *et al* (2009) *The Role of e-Portfolios in Formative and Summative Assessment: Report of the JISC-funded Study*. Centre for Recording Achievement (http://www.jisc.ac.uk/media/documents/programmes/elearning/eportfinalreport.doc).

Index

Compiled by Linda English